Equine Practice

The *In Practice* Handbooks Series

Series Editor: Edward Boden

Past and present members of *In Practice* Editorial Board

Professor J. Armour, Chairman 1979–1989,
Dean, Veterinary Faculty, University of Glasgow

P.B. Clarke
Professor L.B. Jeffcott
J. Richardson
S.A. Hall
Professor M.J. Clarkson
Dr W.M. Allen
B. Martin
K. Urquhart
Dr P.G. Darke
S.D. Gunn
I. Baker
A. Duncan
Professor G.B. Edwards

Titles in print:
Feline Practice
Canine Practice
Equine Practice

Forthcoming titles:
Bovine Practice
Sheep and Goat Practice
Swine Practice

The *In Practice* Handbooks

Equine Practice

Edited by E. Boden
Executive Editor, *In Practice*

Baillière Tindall

LONDON   PHILADELPHIA   TORONTO   SYDNEY   TOKYO

Baillière Tindall   24–28 Oval Road
W.B. Saunders   London NW1 7DX

The Curtis Center
Independence Square West
Philadelphia, PA 19106–3399, USA

55 Horner Avenue
Toronto, Ontario, M8Z 4X6, Canada

Harcourt Brace Jovanovich Group
(Australia) Pty Ltd
30–52 Smidmore Street
Marrickville
NSW 2204, Australia

Harcourt Brace Jovanovich Japan Inc
Ichibancho Central Building,
22–1 Ichibancho
Chiyoda-ku, Tokyo 102, Japan

© 1991 Baillière Tindall

Typeset by Photo·graphics, Honiton, Devon
Printed and bound in Hong Kong by Dah Hua Printing Press Co., Ltd.

A catalogue record for this book is available from the British Library

ISBN 0–7020–1521–0

Contents

Contributors ix

Foreword xi

1 **Vaginal discharge in the mare:** S.W. Ricketts 1
Introduction. Age. Type of mare. Nature of
discharge. Genital tract discharges. Urinary tract
discharges. Conclusions

2 **Caslick's vulvoplasty for the correction of** 27
pneumovagina in mares: S.W. Ricketts and
E.W.M. Curnow
Introduction. Basic principles. Indications. The
operation. Management. Causes of unsatisfactory
results. Alternative approaches

3 **A surgical approach to the cryptorchid horse:** 41
J. Cox
Introduction. Diagnosis. Restraint for
cryptorchidectomy. Inguinal exploration. Supra-
pubic paramedian laparotomy. Locating and
removing the testis. Complications

4 **Air hygiene and equine respiratory disease:** 59
A. Clarke
Introduction. Aetiology. Airborne contaminants of
stables. Air hygiene management. Ventilation of
buildings. Hays. Beddings. Conclusion

5   **Tracheostomy:** P. Dixon   81
    Introduction. Indications for temporary
    tracheostomy. Indications for permanent
    tracheostomy. Surgical anatomy and procedure.
    After care

6   **Grass Sickness:** J.S. Gilmour   97
    Introduction. Diagnosis. Aids to diagnosis. Post-
    mortem findings. Epidemiology and prevention.
    Summary of research

7   **Nasogastric intubation:** K. Urquhart   107
    Introduction. Equipment. Intubation technique.
    Untoward sequelae

8   **Rectal examination of the equine gastrointestinal   115
    tract:** J.M. Hunt
    Introduction. Technique. Routine exploration.
    Specific rectal findings. Significance of rectal
    findings. Additional diagnostic techniques. Rectal
    rupture. Conclusion

9   **Auriculopalpebral and palpebral nerve blocks:**   131
    P. Bedford
    Introduction. Regional analgesia.
    Auriculopalpebral and palpebral nerve block.
    Technique

10 **Nasolacrimal cannulation:** S. Crispin   135
    Introduction. Cannulation

11 **Clinical aspects of equine cardiology:** B. Glazier   143
    Introduction. General examination. Palpation.
    Auscultation of the heart. Heart sounds. Clicks.
    Murmurs. Heart rate. Reliable signs of cardiac
    disease

12 **Forelimb lameness: an approach to diagnosis:**   161
    S.J. Dyson
    Introduction. Where to start. Clinical examination
    at rest. Examination at exercise. Further
    investigation: what to do next. Ultrasonography.
    Diagnosis

13 **Forelimb lameness: diagnosis and treatment:**   185
    S.J. Dyson
    Introduction. Pus in the foot. General trauma with
    secondary infection. Corns. Nail bind or prick.
    The navicular syndrome. Cracked heels. Laminitis.
    Fracture of the distal phalanx. Secondary
    (degenerative) joint disease of the proximal
    interphalangeal joint: ringbone. Sprain of the
    fetlock joint. Periostitis of the second and fourth
    metacarpal bones ("splints"). Strain of the
    superficial or deep digital flexor tendon

14 **Nerve blocks and lameness diagnosis:** S.J. Dyson   211
    Introduction. Prerequisites for diagnosis. Selection
    of local anaesthetic. Equipment and technique.
    Testing the block. Selectivity. Intra-articular
    anaesthesia. Radiography. Nomenclature.
    Desensitization of the palmar third of the
    foot–palmar digital nerve block. Desensitization of
    the foot and pastern – palmar (abaxial sesamoid)
    nerve block. Desensitization of the fetlock and
    pastern – palmar (mid cannon) and palmar
    metacarpal nerve block. Desensitization of the
    metacarpal region – palmar and palmar metacarpal
    (subcarpal) nerve block. Desensitization of the
    carpus and distal limb – ulnar and median nerve
    blocks. Intra-articular analgesia

15 **Problems associated with the interpretation of the**   231
    results of regional and intra-articular anaesthesia:
    S.J. Dyson
    Introduction. Anaesthesia in lameness diagnosis.
    Regional (perineural) anaesthesia. Intra-articular
    anaesthesia. Discussion

16 **Variations in the normal radiographic anatomy of**   243
    equine limbs: S.J. Dyson
    Introduction. Distal (third) phalanx (coffin or
    pedal bone). Summary of standardized
    nomenclature for radiographic projection of the
    limbs. Distal sesamoid (navicular) bone. Middle
    (second) phalanx (short pastern bone). Proximal
    (first) phalanx (long pastern bone).
    Metacarpophalangeal/metatarsophalangeal (fetlock)
    joint. Second, third and fourth
    metacarpal/metatarsal (splint and cannon) bones.
    Carpus. Antebrachium (forearm). Tarsus (hock).
    Stifle. Conclusions

17 **Equine rhabdomyolysis syndrome:** P.A. Harris   265
    Introduction. Clinical signs. Atypical
    myoglobinuria. Diagnosis. Pathophysiology.
    Treatment. Return to work. Prevention.
    Conclusion

18 **Assessment of fitness in the horse:** D. Snow   281
    Introduction. Aims of a training programme.
    Assessment of fitness. Assessment of health

Index   295

Contributors

P.G.C. Bedford Reader in Veterinary Ophthalmology, The Royal Veterinary College, University of London, Hawkshead Campus, Hawkshead Lane, North Mymms, Hatfield, Herts AL9 7TA, UK

A. Clarke Lecturer, Department of Animal Husbandry, University of Bristol, Langford House, Langford, Bristol BS18 7DU, UK

J.E. Cox Senior Lecturer, Division of Equine Studies and Farm Animal Surgery, Department of Veterinary Clinical Science, University of Liverpool, Veterinary Field Station, Leahurst, Neston, South Wirral L64 7TE, UK

S.M. Crispin Lecturer, Department of Veterinary Surgery, School of Veterinary Science, University of Bristol, Langford House, Langford, Bristol BS18 7DU, UK

E.W.M. Curnow Five Acre Farm, West Rudham, King's Lynn, Norfolk PE31 8RW, UK

P.M. Dixon Lecturer, Department of Clinical Veterinary Studies, Royal (Dick) School of Veterinary Studies, Veterinary Field Station, Easter Bush, Nr Roslin, Midlothian EH25 9RG, UK

S.J. Dyson Animal Health Trust, P.O. Box 5, Newmarket, Suffolk CB8 7DW, UK

J.S. Gilmour Animal Diseases Research Association, Moredun Institute, 408 Gilmerton Road, Edinburgh, UK

B. Glazier Department of Veterinary Physiology and Biochemistry, Veterinary College of Ireland, Ballsbridge, Dublin 4, Eire

P.A. Harris The Animal Health Trust, P.O. Box 5, Newmarket, Suffolk CB8 7DW, UK

J.M. Hunt 15 Brook Well, Little Neston, South Wirral, Cheshire L64 0UW, UK

S.W. Ricketts Rossdale & Partners, Veterinary Surgeons, Beaufort Cottage Stables & Laboratories, High Street, Newmarket, Suffolk CB8 8JS, UK

D.H. Snow 31 Mudies Road, St Ives, New South Wales 2075, Australia

K.A. Urquhart 25 Lanark Road, Slateford, Edinburgh EH14 1TG, UK

Foreword

In Practice was started in 1979 as a clinical supplement to *The Veterinary Record*. Its carefully chosen, highly illustrated articles specially commissioned from leaders in their field were aimed specifically at the practitioner. They have proved extremely popular with experienced veterinarians and students alike. The editorial board, chaired for the first 10 years by Professor James Armour, was particularly concerned to emphasize differential diagnosis.

In response to consistent demand, articles from *In Practice*, updated and revised by the authors, are now published in convenient handbook form. Each book deals with a particular species or group of related animals.

E. Boden

CHAPTER 1

Vaginal Discharge in the Mare

SIDNEY W. RICKETTS

INTRODUCTION

Vaginal discharge may indicate genital and, or, urinary abnormality. When making this differential diagnosis, age, type of mare and type of discharge should be considered.

AGE

Genital discharges are less commonly seen in immature and sexually inexperienced mares. If present from birth, congenital or developmental urinary tract abnormalities should be considered. Combinations of genital and urinary discharges may be seen in older broodmares.

TYPE OF MARE

Genital discharges are more commonly seen in broodmares than in mares used for pleasure or performance purposes. Pneumovagina may lead to genital discharge in some immature and sexually inexperienced thoroughbred fillies in training. Vaginal discharges in pregnant mares may indicate urinary, genital, fetoplacental or vaginal abnormality. Transient vaginal discharge is commonly seen immediately post partum, but persistent discharge may indicate parturient trauma and, or, endometritis with delayed uterine involution.

NATURE OF DISCHARGE

Genital discharges are usually thick, tenacious, grey/cream/yellow/brownish in colour, often visible at the ventral commissure of the vulval lips, sometimes matted in the tail and smeared on either side of the buttocks at that level and are seldom irritant to the perineal skin (Fig. 1.1). Urinary tract discharges are usually thinner, less tenacious, clearer and are irritant to the local skin, often "scalding" the ventral commissure of the vulva and the medial aspects of the thighs (Fig. 1.2). Where the tail is soaked with urine, concomitant caudal neuropathy/paresis should be considered.

Blood staining or haemorrhagic discharge is more frequently

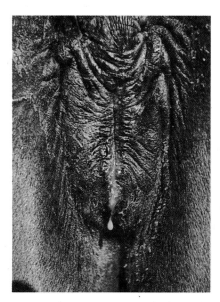

Fig. 1.1
Example of vaginal discharge of genital origin.

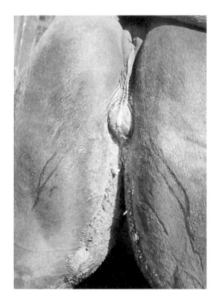

Fig. 1.2
Example of vaginal discharge of urinary origin. Note "scalding".

seen in urinary than genital abnormality, but in late pregnant mares vaginal haemorrhage may indicate premature placental separation or vaginal varicose vein damage. In post parturient mares, haemorrhagic vaginal discharge may been seen during the involuntary period, indicating that significant uteroplacental haemorrhage occurred at placental separation.

GENITAL TRACT DISCHARGES

VAGINITIS/CERVICITIS

Pneumovagina, i.e. the aspiration of air into the vagina, is the most common cause of vaginitis/cervicitis in thoroughbred broodmares and sometimes fillies in training. Genetic influences, with selection for racing performance alone, appear to have resulted in an ever increasing number of mares with the well-known unsatisfactory perineal conformation which predisposes to this condition.

Ideally, the vulva should be situated in a vertical line beneath the anus, with its upper commissure at the level of the pelvic brim. There are then three functional "seals" (vulval, vestibular and cervical) between the external environment and the uterine lumen. Where the vulva slopes caudally from beneath the anus and, or, the upper commissure is above the pelvic brim, the vulval and vestibular seals are compromised. They no longer prevent air, contaminated with environmental debris and microorganisms, from being aspirated into the vagina when the mare moves, resulting in a vaginitis, which may produce a vulval discharge. Perineal or environmental microorganisms such as *Streptococcus zooepidemicus*, *Escherichia coli*, *Staphylococcus aureus* and *Staph. albus* are common opportunist pathogens.

In fillies in training, pneumovagina may occur because of immature vulval and perineal fat pad development, which may result in a concave, sloping vulva. There is sometimes spontaneous improvement with maturity and pregnancy. Later, after repeated pregnancy and with increasing age and abdominal girth, the anus may displace in a cranial direction. This displacement pulls the upper commissure of the vulva forward in a convex slope, over the pelvic brim. This results not only in vulval and vestibular seal incompetence and pneumovagina but allows faeces to drop into the vestibule, complicating the vaginitis (Fig. 1.3). Vaginitis progresses to cervicitis and when the mare comes into oestrus the cervical seal is lost and endometritis, and sometimes pneumouterus, occurs.

Vaginoscopy reveals an inflamed vagina and cervix, sometimes with grey or cream/yellow discharge and occasionally small air bubbles at the cervix. Cytological examination of the discharge reveals large numbers of polymorphonuclear leucocytes, in varying stages of degeneration, some exhibiting active phagocytosis of bacteria and debris. Bacteriological culture of the discharge usually reveals a mixed growth of organisms, as discussed above. Treatment is by Caslick's vulvoplasty operation or Pouret's perineal reconstruction.

CASLICK'S VULVOPLASTY

Caslick's vulvoplasty operation is performed under local infiltration anaesthesia, with the mare restrained in the standing position. After removal of the mucosa on both sides,

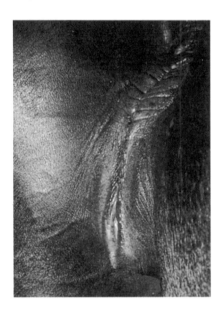

Fig. 1.3
Vulva of an aged mare with "convex" sloping
conformation, causing pneumovagina and faecal
soiling of the vestibule.

the vulval lips are sutured together from the level of the pelvic
brim to the upper commissure (Fig. 1.4). This technique alone
will usually result in a resolution of the vaginitis/cervicitis,
but concurrent systemic antimicrobial medication may be
administered, if indicated. Where endometritis is also present,
this may require specific treatment.

Perineal conformation, and the indication for surgical treatment, may be judged by visual inspection of the vulval slope
in relation to the anus and by digitally defining the level of
the pelvis in relation to the upper commissure of the vulva.
Some mares in oestrus appear to require vulval surgery,
but examination during dioestrus shows that competent
conformation has been restored. Indiscriminate and excessive
vulval surgery is to be deplored, especially in young healthy
mares, where repeated episiotomy and surgical repair for
mating and foaling can provide healing difficulties which may
jeopardize the future breeding career of the mare. Veterinary
surgeons must resist pressures from some trainers and owners
who appear to look upon "the Caslick" as a panacea for all
forms of performance and reproductive failure.

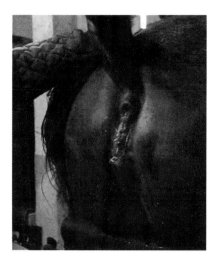

Fig. 1.4
Caslick's vulvoplasty operation – the vulval lips
have been sutured to the level of the pelvis.

POURET'S PERINEAL RECONSTRUCTION

Pouret's perineal reconstruction operation is an alternative treatment to Caslick's vulvoplasty designed to avoid the narrowing of the vulval aperture. With the mare tranquillized and restrained in the standing position, preferably in stocks, an epidural anaesthetic is administered. Local anaesthetic solution is infiltrated under the perineal skin and into the rectovaginal shelf. A horizontal, mid-perineal skin incision is then made midway between the anus and the upper commissure of the vulva, and the subcutaneous fascia is separated. The rectovaginal shelf is then separated by blunt and sharp dissection, cranially to the peritoneal reflection. This allows the rectum and anus to migrate cranially, independent of the vagina and vulva. The latter is then able to return to a more caudal and vertical position. The skin wound is sutured vertically or with a 'T' shaped closure to maximize the horizontal shelf formed between the anus and the vulva (Fig. 1.5).

Currently, this technique is used mostly for older mares who have previously undergone Caslick's operation and who require more radical surgery. It remains to be seen if Pouret's operation alone can be successfully used on younger mares as a "first choice".

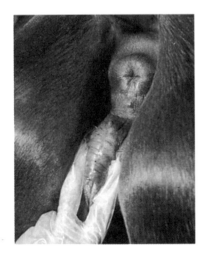

Fig. 1.5
Pouret's perineal reconstruction operation healed –
the rectovaginal shelf has been separated, forming
a horizontal shelf between the anus and the more
caudal and vertical vulva. This mare had previously
undergone a Caslick's vulvoplasty.

ENDOMETRITIS

Pneumovagina can cause vaginal discharge associated with vaginitis and cervicitis. During oestrus the cervix becomes moist, pink and relaxed, allowing the vaginitis and cervicitis to ascend to endometritis. Environmental opportunist microorganisms gain access to the uterine lumen, invade the inflamed endometrium and may produce a purulent discharge which may vary in degree from being detectable only on cytological or histological examination, to frank pyometra (Fig. 1.6).

Endometritis may follow cervical or rectovaginal damage. Cervical closure, during dioestrus, is necessary to seal the uterine lumen from the vaginal and external environment. Cervical damage may occur during mating, or more commonly

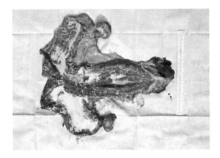

Fig. 1.6
Pyometra – opened necropsy uterus.

during foaling, often associated with dystocia. Cervical adhesions trap inflammatory exudate, which is intermittently released, producing a vulval discharge. Rectovaginal injury occasionally occurs at parturition, producing either a fistula or a third degree perineal laceration, allowing faecal contamination of the vagina and uterus (Fig. 1.7). Cervical and rectovaginal surgery is usually performed under epidural anaesthesia, with the mare standing restrained, ideally, in stocks. Details of these specialized surgical techniques may be obtained from the references list.

All mares produce an acute endometritis following mating. The cervix relaxes during oestrus, allowing ejaculation into the uterine lumen. The uterine lumen is contaminated with environmental, penile and perineal microorganisms and debris, in addition to semen. At 24–48 h after mating, all mares show cytological evidence of acute endometritis and in some cases this may be severe enough to produce a visible vulval discharge. Most mares, without pneumovagina, cervical or rectovaginal damage, have efficient local immunological defence mechanisms which resolve the endometritis by 72–96 h.

As yet the precise details of these mechanisms are incom-

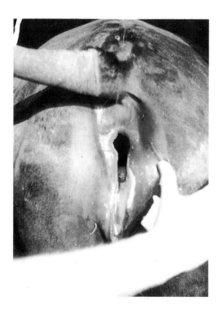

Fig. 1.7
Healed third degree perineal laceration, sustained at parturition, allowing faecal soiling of the vagina.

pletely understood, but it is recognized that efficient phagocytosis by mobilized uterine luminal leucocytes is an essential
feature (Fig. 1.8). In some, usually older, multiparous mares
the defence mechanisms fail, resulting in persistent acute post
coital endometritis. These mares may persistently discharge
after mating or, more usually, they may produce a vulval
discharge at 10–15 days after mating, when the endometritis
causes premature endogenous prostaglandin release and luteolysis, resulting in early return to oestrus and cervical relaxation.

DIAGNOSIS

Diagnosis of endometritis can be made by vaginoscopic
examination where purulent material can be seen discharging
through the cervix. A visible discharge is not always present
and the cytological examination of an endometrial smear,
taken via a vaginoscope through the open oestrous cervix, is
a simple, rapid diagnostic aid. The presence of endometrial
epithelial cells defines a representative smear (Fig. 1.9) and
the presence of polymorphonuclear leucocytes defines an acute
endometritis (Fig. 1.10). The mare, unlike some other species,
does not have an oestral "leucocytic tide". In mares at first
post partum oestrus ("foal-heat"), and in maiden mares at first
oestrus after winter anoestrus, some degenerate polymorphonuclear leucocytes (less than 5%) may be acceptable in
association with the clearance of accumulated luminal
secretions and the products of repair processes, otherwise no
polymorphonuclear leucocytes should be seen in an oestral
endometrial smear.

Bacterial infection may be confirmed and defined by a

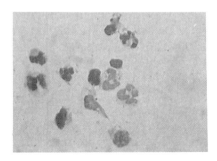

Fig. 1.8
Endometrial smear showing Gram-negative
coccobacilli (*Taylorella equigenitalis*) engulfed in
active polymorphonuclear phagocytes. Gram's
stain × 1600.

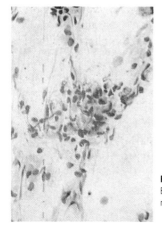

Fig. 1.9
Endometrial epithelial cells in smear taken from a normal oestral
mare. Pollack's trichrome × 630.

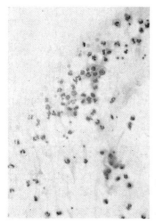

Fig. 1.10
Endometrial epithelial cells and polymorphonuclear leucocytes in
smear taken from an oestral mare with acute endometritis. Pollack's
Trichrome × 630.

Gram's stained smear and by the culture of a concurrently taken
endometrial swab sample. The significance of bacteriological
growth from such samples can only be accurately assessed in
the light of cytological results, because of the technical
problems of obtaining swab samples uncontaminated with
mucosal surface contaminants or commensals, even when
elaborate guarded swabbing techniques are attempted. As
discussed above, *Strep. zooepidemicus, E. coli, Staph. aureus*
and *Staph. albus* are the common opportunist pathogens
isolated from endometritis cases. Other environmental and
perineal contaminants, such as *Corynebacterium* species,

Anthracoides species, *Strep. faecalis, Proteus* species, *Entero-bacter aerogenes,* and anaerobes such as *Bacteroides fragilis, Clostridium perfringens, Cl. mortiferum, Peptococcus* species, and *Peptostreptococcus* species, may gain access to the uterus and become associated with endometritis, usually in mixed infections.

Klebsiella pneumoniae (capsule types 1, 2 and 5), some strains of *Pseudomonas aeruginosa* (not yet distinguishable by laboratory tests) and the contagious metritis microaerophilic coccobacillus *Taylorella equigenitalis* have been isolated in venereal endometritis, resulting in epidemic vaginal discharge after mating. These organisms, which are not commonly environmental or perineal contaminants, are usually passed from carrier mare to stallion where they colonize the penile and preputial smegma, before being mechanically passed to other mares at mating. They appear able to infect mares with competent and incompetent local uterine defence mechanisms.

Concurrent endometrial swab and smear examinations are the most practical and useful techniques for the diagnosis of acute endometritis in mares, before mating. For a more detailed definition of the nature and severity of the endometritis, the histological examination of a biopsy specimen is required. Endometrial biopsy specimens may be obtained, using special basket-jawed forceps, simply and safely in any non-pregnant mare. Polymorphonuclear leucocyte infiltrations indicate acute endometritis (Fig. 1.11), whereas mononuclear cell infiltrations, glandular degenerative changes and stromal fibrosis are features of chronic endometritis (Figs 1.12 and 1.13).

Mixed pathology is commonly seen in non-pregnant, multiparous brood mares and histopathological changes must be carefully interpreted with respect to age and breeding history. In addition to age and cyclic histological changes, the repeated challenge of semen and associated environmental contamination, pregnancy, parturition and involution leads to progressive histopathological changes which are unavoidable to a degree which must be assessed in individual cases.

TREATMENT

Treatment for acute bacterial endometritis is based on the use of specific antibacterial drugs, removal of predisposing causes,

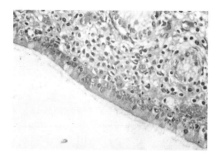

Fig. 1.11 Endometrial biopsy specimen of a case of acute endometritis. Polymorphonuclear leucocytes migrating through the superficial stroma and luminal epithelium on their way to the uterine lumen. Haematoxylin and eosin × 630.

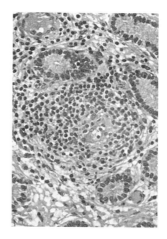

Fig. 1.12 Endometrial biopsy specimen of a case of chronic infiltrative endometritis. Dense periglandular mononuclear cell infiltration. Haematoxylin and eosin × 630.

promotion of drainage where there is uterine discharge or pyometra and the use of techniques which may aid compromised local defence mechanisms.

Specific antibacterial drugs (based on the results of in vitro sensitivity tests), may be used systemically and, or, locally.

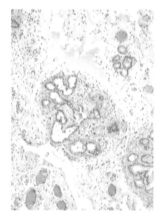

Fig. 1.13
Endometrial biopsy specimen of a case of chronic degenerative
endometritis. Glandular "nest" degeneration, associated with dense,
stromal fibrosis. Haematoxylin and eosin × 160.

Experience suggests that systemic treatment alone is seldom
effective. Few commercially available antibiotic preparations
are manufactured with intrauterine use in mind and many
are unsuitable in that they are irritant (e.g. tetracyclines), leave
insoluble remnants (e.g. ampicillin) or have insoluble or
irritant vehicles (e.g. all pessary and oil based preparations).
Experience suggests that a water soluble mixture of neomycin
(1 g), polymixin B (40000 iu) and furaltadone (600 mg) (Intrauterine wash; Univet), with or without crystalline benzylpenicillin (5 mega) (Crystapen; Glaxovet), installed into the uterus
via a sterile catheter or insemination pipette, daily for 3–5
days, is a successful treatment for a wide range of bacterial
endometritis cases and may be used confidently as a "first
choice" treatment. Untoward sequelae such as local inflammation, mycotic or *Pseudomonas* species overgrowth, reported
with some intrauterine antibiotic therapy, have been rarely
reported with this antibiotic mixture, probably because of its
non-irritant, no residue, water soluble properties. Although
more specific treatment may be considered preferable in
individual cases, bacteriological surveys suggest that mixed
infections, with aerobic and sometimes anaerobic organisms,
are often present and the 'broad spectrum' approach is
frequently indicated. *B. fragilis* is sensitive to furaltadone and
most other anaerobes are sensitive to penicillin.

In some cases, an indwelling uterine infuser (catheter)
(Arnolds) provides an efficient means of administering once
or twice daily infusions. The catheter is introduced through

the cervix and the intrauterine device is extruded in the caudal uterine body. The distal end of the catheter is fixed, over loosely applied stay sutures, to the vulvo-buttock junction. Intrauterine medication may be infused via a syringe and 16 gauge needle, before replacing a tight fitting cap. Providing the cervix retains tone, i.e. the mare does not come into oestrus during a course of treatment, the catheters remain in place. If stay sutures are tied tightly to the perineal skin, this may cause irritation and the mare may rub the catheter out. The catheter can be removed at the end of a course of treatment by removing the stay sutures and applying gentle traction to the catheter.

Antibacterial treatment for endometritis will only be temporarily successful if predisposing causes, such as pneumovagina, cervical or rectovaginal damage, remain untreated. These must be corrected, if possible, before or at the same time as antibiotic treatment.

Failure of uterine defence mechanisms

In persistent acute endometritis cases, where structural predisposing factors cannot be identified, it is assumed that the mare's natural uterine defence mechanisms have failed. Research has shown that although large numbers of polymorphonuclear leucocytes are mobilized in the endometrium and migrate into the uterine lumen, as in normal mares, these polymorphonuclear leucocytes have depressed phagocytic capacity. The lesion appears to be at the level of bacterial opsonization and as complement is an essential component of the opsonization "cascade" reaction, a deficiency or inactivation of uterine complement may be involved. In vitro studies involving the addition of homologous plasma (as a source of complement) have resulted in improved phagocytosis and in vivo studies with uterine plasma treatments have been encouraging. Blood can be collected from the mare, during oestrus if possible, in vacuum packs (Travenol Laboratories, available from Arnolds) and, on standing, the erythrocytes will settle out within two to three hours. The plasma can then be transferred into 150 ml transfer packs (Travenol), which can be refrigerated overnight or frozen if longer storage is required. Before use the plasma is warmed to 38°C. Three to six daily intrauterine infusions of plasma, with or without antibiotic treatment, have been successful in resolving persistent acute endometritis in individual cases. Further research, clinical experience and time will determine if this approach is the fundamental answer to such a complex problem.

Pyometra

In cases of endometritis with accumulated uterine discharge/secretions or in cases of frank pyometra, drainage of the accumulated material is essential. Ultrasound echography, using a real-time linear array 3.5 or 5.0 MHz transrectal probe, provides an excellent means of differential diagnosis for cases of pyometra or uterine fluid accumulation (Fig. 1.14). Where cervical closure prevents drainage, endogenous prostaglandin treatment should cause luteolysis followed by cervical relaxation. The cervix should be examined digitally for luminal adhesions, which may prevent drainage. If found, adhesions should be broken down by careful digital manipulation and hydrocortisone and antibiotic ointment (2% sodium fusidate and 1% hydrocortisone acetate, Fucidin-H; Leo Laboratories)

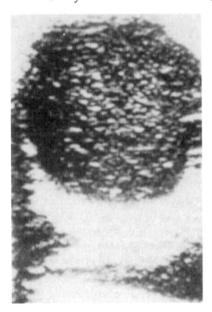

Fig. 1.14
Pyometra. Ultrasound scan photograph showing cross section of uterine horn containing highly particular (echogenic) fluid.

applied daily for 7–10 days to promote smooth healing and to inhibit reformation.

Large volume uterine irrigation

In mares with pendulous uteri, luminal contents may pool in the ventral areas, preventing natural drainage. Repeated active drainage of the luminal contents may be indicated. This may be achieved via an extended, two-way, size 30 French Foley catheter (Franklin Medical) through which 3–4 litres of saline solution can be infused, the uterus massaged per rectum, if indicated, and then the saline allowed to flow out. Repeated uterine flushings are made until the saline outflow becomes visibly clear and cytological examinations reveal the flushings to be free of polymorphonuclear leucocytes. In such mares, ventral uterine "dilations" may be caused by local chronic endometrial and sometimes myometrial damage resulting in loss of endometrial folds and muscular stretching. There is no consistently successful treatment for this condition but in some cases, repeated irrigations with hot (45–50°C) saline solution may improve the overall tone of the uterus, reducing the effect of the dilatations. The breeding prognosis in these cases is always guarded.

Similar treatment may be used for cases of pyometra. Alternatively, two stomach tubes may be placed through the cervix, one into a uterine horn and the other just inside the cervix. Large volumes of saline, or in these cases tap water, may be flushed through the tube in the uterine horn and out of the tube at the cervix. The outflow tube is periodically blocked to distend the uterus before allowing outflow to continue. Mild antiseptic solutions, for example povidone iodine (2%), are sometimes used but the distention and flushing action is thought to be most important. Hydrogen peroxide (2% w/v) may help in the removal of necrotic tissue and debris.

In cases of pyometra there is usually a predisposing factor or factors involved, such as cervical damage or chronic *Ps. aeruginosa* or mycotic infection. These must be identified and treated if possible. The breeding prognosis for pyometra cases is always very poor and most cases recur spontaneously or following mating, even where minimal contamination techniques are used.

Minimal contamination mating techniques

In all mares where acute endometritis has been treated and depressed local immune mechanisms are suspected, prophylactic techniques are recommended to reduce the risk of recurrence following mating. The mare is mated once only, just before ovulation of a palpably normal mature ovarian follicle. As all mares produce an acute endometritis following mating, another mating at 2–3 days after the first is clearly contraindicated. Artificial insemination with washed, antibiotic-treated and extended semen is the ideal method of reducing the bacterial content of the semen introduced into the uterus, but in thoroughbred mares, this technique is precluded by registration requirements. As a "next best" approach, a semen extender (containing antibiotics) (Table 1.1), warmed to 38°C, is instilled into the uterus of the mare just before natural mating, reducing the bacterial content of the semen after ejaculation.

Another approach is to irrigate the mare's uterus, with antibiotics and, or, homologous plasma, 24–48 h after mating, while the fertilized ovum, if present, is in the fallopian tube. Combinations of these techniques have been used in some particularly intractable cases. Subjective impressions are that these techniques are of real value in the management of persistent endometritis cases, but objective, critically con-

Table 1.1 Recipe for semen extender suitable for precoital use, as part of a minimal contamination breeding technique. After Kenney *et al.*, 1975.

Instant, low fat, dry skim milk (Marvel)	2·5 g
Gelatin, powdered, no flavour or sugar	0·5 g
Glucose	5·0 g
Penicillin, crystalline	300 mg
Streptomycin, crystalline	300 mg
Water, sterile	100 ml

trolled studies are difficult if not impossible to arrange for such a complex multifactorial problem.

PLACENTITIS

Chronic placentitis may cause vaginal discharge in late pregnant mares. Haematogenous or low grade uterine infections usually result in early embryonic or fetal death and resorption or abortion without prior discharge. Ascending infections may occur, via the cervix, during late pregnancy. Pneumovagina, vaginal urine pooling or cervical damage are common predisposing factors and the concomitant vaginitis/cervicitis results in visible discharge. Mixed bacterial infections and sometimes fungal infections are involved. In some cases abortion may occur but in others a small impoverished premature or dysmature foal may be born, with gross evidence of a body placentitis which radiates from the area of the cervical star (Fig. 1.15)

For cases of placentitis, prevention is much better than cure. Good hygienic studfarm management with the treatment and prevention of endometritis, where indicated, should maintain the incidence of placentitis at low levels. Once discharge is visible and the causal organism identified and sensitivity tests performed, treatment may be attempted by the use of systemic antimicrobial drugs. Placental pathology will, however, remain and facilities for neonatal critical care should be prepared for use if necessary.

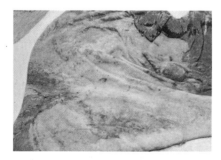

Fig. 1.15
Chronic mycotic placentitis. Body of placenta with thick grey/yellow diphthitic membrane emanating from the area of the cervical star.

PREMATURE PLACENTAL SEPARATION

This is an unusual condition which may result in a haemor-rhagic vaginal discharge at or near term. Diagnosis may be made by vaginoscopic examination, where blood may be seen discharging through a relaxing cervix. This is a fetal life-threatening condition and is an indication for induction of parturition (5 iu oxytocin intravenously) if satisfactory criteria are met to suggest readiness for birth. The mare should be over 340 days gestation and should have colostrum in its udder. The biochemical analysis of mammary secretions may help where gross examinations are not straight forward. Analyses should reveal calcium at greater than 12.0 mmol/l, sodium at greater than 30 mmol/l and potassium at greater than 20 mmol/l.

Rapid "strip" tests, based on water hardness testing kits, provide helpful results in emergency situations. Facilities for neonatal critical care should be prepared for use if necessary.

VESTIBULAR VARICOSE VEINS

Premature placental separation must be differentiated from the intermittent, late gestational haemorrhagic vaginal discharge which occurs in some mares associated with dorsal vestibular varicose veins. This condition, although worrying to the owner, is usually of no consequence to the mare or its pregnancy and seldom requires treatment. Haemostasis by electrocautery and surgical ligation has been reported.

URINARY TRACT DISCHARGES

ECTOPIC URETER

Congenital anatomical abnormalities of the ureteral exits are rare in horses. Ectopic ureters may bypass bladder sphincter control, leading to urinary incontinence (Fig. 1.16). There is a persistent vaginal urine discharge, present from birth, which causes persistent scalding of the hindlimb.

Ureteral ectopia may be confirmed by placing a simple dye, such as methylene blue, into the bladder by catheter and observing unstained urine continue to dribble from the vulva until voluntary urination, or frusemide stimulated urination, empties the bladder and voids the dye (Fig. 1.17). If necessary, further confirmation may be obtained using contrast radiography. Attempts at surgical correction are possible but are technically difficult and are seldom considered appropriate.

URETHRITIS

Primary urethritis is uncommon in mares, but may be seen secondarily to cystitis.

CYSTITIS/URINARY INCONTINENCE

Cystitis is uncommon in mares. It seldom causes vaginal discharge unless associated with vesicular calculi, polyps or tumours which may act as "ball-valves", leading to urine retention and overflow incontinence which scalds the hind legs (Fig. 1.18). Urinary incontinence may also occur following damage to the neurological innervation to the bladder. This may be seen with equine herpesvirus 1 posterior paresis and neuritis of the cauda equina. Overflow urinary incontinence occurs, soaking the paralysed tail and scalding the hindlimbs.

Urine analysis reveals the presence of leucocytes and sometimes erythrocytes. These cells and epithelial debris will produce positive protein and sometimes blood and haemoglobin reactions. Bacteria and sometimes yeasts may be seen on

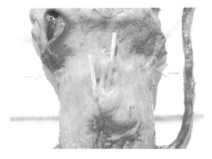

Fig. 1.16
Congenital ureteral ectopia. Necropsy specimen showing level of bladder neck (arrows) with asymmetrical ureteral outlets.

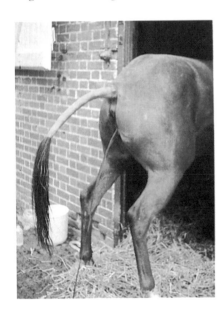

Fig. 1.17
Congenital ureteral ectopia. Filly urinating methylene
blue stained urine from bladder after frusemide
treatment. Before treatment, clear urine had
dribbled from the vulva after the dye had been
placed in the bladder by catheter.

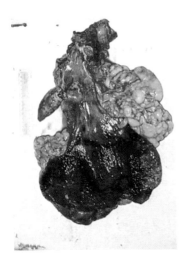

Fig. 1.18
Necropsy specimen showing pedunculated
fibroepithelial polyp in the neck of the bladder of a
pony mare previously showing signs of "overflow"
urinary incontinence and retention cystitis.

microscopic examination. The significance of microorganisms may be unclear, but where isolated in pure culture from urine samples obtained by catheter, using aseptic techniques and where leucocytes are present in significant numbers, a bacterial or mycotic cystitis may be diagnosed. The specific gravity may be elevated and the pH, which varies with diet, may be outside the normal range. Horses receiving high concentrate performance diets have a urine pH of 6.0–7.2 whereas horses at grass have a urine pH of 7.6–8.8.

Calcium carbonate crystals, and sometimes urate and oxalate crystals, are a normal feature of equine urine samples and do not necessarily indicate calculus formation. Vesicular calculi may be either sabulous, where a sand-like mass of small calculi pack down in the ventral aspect of the bladder, eventually becoming large enough to embarrass urine outflow, or discrete, where one or more large formed calculi form (Fig. 1.19). Rectal palpation may reveal the presence of calculi and, if large and discrete, their surface may be palpated digitally via the urethra, while being held in the neck of the bladder by the other hand, per rectum. "Ball-valve" lesions often cause distention of the bladder with urine, which may cause colic. Passage of a urethral catheter into the bladder may allow the operator to appreciate the "feel" of the lesion, transmitted through the catheter and will displace the lesion cranially, allowing urine to escape through the catheter.

Vesicular endoscopy is a simple and very useful technique in the mare. A clear view of the lumen of the bladder, its contents, the appearance of the epithelial lining and the outlets of the ureters may be obtained. However, where there is a large, discrete, lumen-occupying lesion, endoscopy may not provide a view which is clear enough to define the lesion and

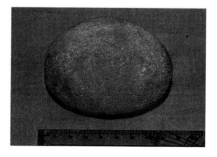

Fig. 1.19
Discrete calcium carbonate and phosphate vesicular calculus removed digitally via the urethra from a sedated mare previously showing signs of "overflow" urinary incontinence and retention cystitis.

rectal palpation may be more rewarding.

Ultrasound echography provides a simple technique which can define the contents of the bladder. Good contrast is obtained between fluid urine (black) and tissue or particulate material (white). Crystals produce a "scintillating" or "snow-storm" appearance, the density of which is proportional to their concentration. Polyps or tumours may contrast white against the darker urine and large calculi may have a dense, white, lamellar structure, definable at the surface.

Neurological examinations will reveal paralysis of the tail and anus and posterior paresis causing ataxia, in equine herpesvirus 1 infection and neuritis of the cauda equina. Overflow incontinence and cystitis, in these cases, are secondary phenomena and may resolve if the primary neurological signs respond to early treatment. If there is no neurological improvement, euthanasia is indicated.

Treatment of bacterial or mycotic cystitis, with or without the presence of small or sabulous calculi, may be attempted by repeated flushing of the bladder with sterile saline solution via a large bore urethral catheter, until the flushings appear clear and particle free. If microorganisms are involved, appropriate non-irritant antibiotic or antifungal medication may be added. If the urine pH is high and sabulous calcium carbonate calculi are present, acidification of the urine by altering the diet (increasing concentrates, reducing access to grass) and feeding hexamine may be helpful.

Polyps, tumours or calculi may require surgical removal by cystotomy under general anaesthesia. However, it may be possible to remove even relatively large free calculi, by careful and patient digital manipulation, via the urethra of a cooperative, sedate mare. Following removal of such lesions the bladder should be thoroughly flushed with sterile saline solution with added antimicrobial medication where appropriate.

Following removal of the predisposing cause (benign vesicular lesions and, or, microbial infection), urinary incontinence and vaginal discharge usually resolves quite quickly.

VAGINAL URINE POOLING

This condition may occur intermittently or persistently, resulting in overflow incontinence and urine scalding of the ventral vulva and medial thighs. Intermittent cases are sometimes seen post partum during the immediate uterine involutionary period or in cases of delayed post partum uterine involution, often associated with acute endometritis. The enlarged and pendulous uterus drags the vagina in a cranioventral direction, displacing the urethral opening to the pelvic brim and allowing "splashback" during urination. Vaginoscopic examination reveals a pool of urine in the cranial vagina and the cervix appearing displaced cranioventrally.

Treatment is by the promotion of uterine involution (60 iu oxytocin in 500 ml saline by intravenous drip) and the concomitant treatment of acute endometritis, where present, as described below. Following successful treatment of the predisposing factors, the vaginal urine pooling usually resolves.

Persistent cases usually occur in older mares with poor perineal conformation. Stretching of the abdominal muscles and the development of a pendulous uterus results in a cranioventral displacement of the intestines, anus and vagina. The urethral opening is displaced over the pelvic brim, preventing complete urine evacuation.

Treatment is by the Pouret perineal reconstruction operation which separates the anus and rectum from the vulva and vagina, allowing the urethral opening to return to its normal position. Where the uterus is pendulous, associated with endometritis, lymphatic pooling, pyometra or fluid accumulation, specific treatment should be attempted. Plastic surgical techniques, which extend the urethral opening in a caudal direction, have been described and details may be obtained from the reference list. These latter techniques do not attempt to treat the predisposing causes.

CONCLUSIONS

Vaginal discharge is but a sign of genital and, or, urinary disease and specific diagnosis of the primary and predisposing abnormalities is a prerequisite for successful treatment.

REFERENCES AND FURTHER READING

Asbury, A. C. (1984) *Theriogenology* **21**, 397.

Hackett, R. P., Vaughan, J. T. & Tennant, B. C. (1982). Diseases of the urinary bladder In *Equine Medicine & Surgery*, 3rd edn p. 912 (Eds R. A. Mansmann, E.S. McAllister and P. W. Pratt). Santa Barbara, California, American Veterinary Publications.

Kenney, R. M., Bergman, R. V. Cooper, W. L. & Morse, G. W. (1975). Minimal contamination techniques for breeding mares: technique and preliminary findings. In *Proceedings of the 21st Annual Convention of the American Association of Equine Practitioners*, p. 327.

Pouret, E. J. M. (1982) *Equine Veterinary Journal* **14**, 249.

Ricketts, S. W. (1981) *Veterinary Record* **108**, 52.

Rossdale, P. D. & Ricketts, S. W. (1980). *Equine Studfarm Medicine* 2nd edn. London, Baillière Tindall.

Walker, D. F. & Vaughan, J. T. (1980). *Bovine and Equine Urogenital Surgery*, Philadelphia, Lea & Febiger.

Wingfield Digby, N. J. & Ricketts, S. W. (1982) *Journal of Reproduction and Fertility* Supplement **32**, 181.

CHAPTER 2

Caslick's Vulvoplasty for the Correction of Pneumovagina in Mares

SIDNEY W. RICKETTS AND EUAN W. M. CURNOW

INTRODUCTION

In 1937, Caslick described deformities in the perineal conformation of some thoroughbred mares, which could cause
pneumovagina and sometimes faecal contamination of the
vestibule, leading to cervicitis, endometritis and subfertility.
He described a correcting vulvoplasty operation which reduced
the vulval aperture. This operation became known universally
as the "Caslick" operation. It was a "milestone" in equine
gynaecology and it remains an invaluable aid to equine
fertility.

BASIC PRINCIPLES

The equine genitalia, from the vulva to the tips of the uterine
horns, form a continuous tube. The uterus, which must
support sperm transport, reception of the fertilized ovum and
maintenance of pregnancy to full term, must be protected
from the microbial ecosystems of the external genitalia and

the general environment of the horse.

The "normal" mare has three functional seals which form a barrier between the external environment and the uterine lumen, i.e. the vulva, the vestibulo-vaginal and the cervix. During oestrus, the vulva and cervix relax and so maintenance of uterine sterility depends on the integrity of the vestibulo-vaginal seal (see Fig. 2.1). Optimal conformation is one in which the vulval lips are in the vertical plane and 80% of their length is below the level of the pelvic brim, i.e. the ischium.

Changes in the normal relationship of perineal structures occur with advancing age and multiparity as the pelvic and abdominal ligaments and muscles lose their effectiveness (see Fig. 2.2). Where the vulva is high in relation to the pelvic brim, the vestibular seal may be compromised and pneumovagina may occur as the mare walks. Where the vulva slopes ventro-caudally and away from a "sunken" anus, pneumovagina is complicated by faecal contamination, as faeces fall into the vestibule. Where the vestibule and urethral opening are displaced cranially, urovagina may occur.

Pneumovagina and, or, urovagina lead to vaginitis, cervictis and endometritis, resulting in subfertility.

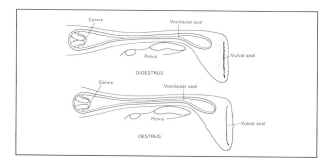

Fig. 2.1 Lateral view of the normal anatomical relationships between the posterior genitalia and the ischium, showing three functional seals between the uterus and the environment. During dioestrus the cervix is closed; the vulval and vestibulo-vaginal seals are effective. During oestrus the cervix and vulva are relaxed; the vestibular seal is penetrated at coitus, leaving natural endometrial immune defence mechanisms to maintain genital health. (From Rossdale and Ricketts 1980.)

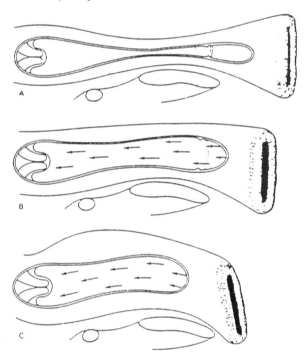

Fig. 2.2 View as in Figure 2.1, but for a dioestrous mare with unsatisfactory perineal conformation. (From Rossdale and Ricketts 1980.) (A) The ischium is low in relation to the vulva, producing an ineffective vestibular seal. The vulva is closed so the cervix is not challenged until the mare is in oestrus. (B) As in (A) but an incompetent vulva allows penumovagina during dioestrus and oestrus. (C) As in (B), further aggravated by a sloping vulva which allows faecal contamination.

INDICATIONS

The perineal conformation of any mare which fails to conceive, after mating with a known fertile stallion, should be investigated.

A gloved finger is passed horizontally through the vulval lips, to rest on the pelvic brim. If this level is significantly below the upper vulval commissure and especially where the vulva above slopes ventro-caudally away from the anus, the perineal shape has the potential to produce pneumovagina. Faecal contamination of the vestibule can be identified by digitally parting the vulval lips.

Pneumovagina may be confirmed by vaginoscopic examination. There may be visual evidence of vaginal inflammation and, occasionally, purulent material and, or, small bubbles of air at the cervix. Cervicitis and endometritis can be confirmed by the cytological identification of polymorphonuclear leucocytes in smear samples.

Pascoe (1979) designed an instrument to measure the effective length (L) (cm) and angle of declination (A) of the vulva from which to calculate a "Caslick Index" (L × A). This may provide a more objective assessment of the need to operate on mares not showing the classic symptoms of pneumovagina. Mares with an index of less than 150 had a significantly higher pregnancy rate than those with a higher index and L showed a significant increase with age.

As with any surgical procedure, the Caslick operation should only be performed where there are clear indications for its need. There has been a tendency in recent years to abuse the operation, with unnecessary or excessively extensive surgery being performed, in some cases leading to managerial and gynaecological problems. Accurate diagnosis of pneumovagina, i.e. the indication for corrective surgery, is, as always, a prerequisite.

THE OPERATION

RESTRAINT

Ideally, the mare is restrained, bridled, in stocks. Where mare temperament and lay assistance is satisfactory, however, this operation can be performed with the mare restrained by bridle in her stable, with her buttocks positioned at the door frame. It is the responsibility of the surgeon to ensure the safety of the mare, lay assistants and himself, in each individual case.

The operation is frequently performed under local anaesthesia alone, but tranquillization may be a valuable aid to technique and safety in some cases. We have found detomidine hydrochloride (8 mg/kg intravenously) (Domosedan; Smith Kline Animal Health) to be particularly useful as, in addition to its analgesic effects, it helps to produce an immobile patient. Recently the combination of detomidine hydrochloride (8 mg/kg, i.e. 0.4 ml, intravenously) and butorphanol (1 µg/kg, i.e. 1.0 ml, intravenously) (Torbugesic; C-Vet) has been found to be capable of rendering even most aggressive mares immobile.

PREPARATION

Tetanus immune status is supplemented as necessary. In most cases, systemic antibacterial treatment is not indicated but where it is, a loading dose should be given before surgery.

The mare's tail should be bandaged and held to one side by an assistant. The perineum should be thoroughly washed with warm water to provide a clean surgical site (Fig. 2.3). The repeated use of antiseptic solutions in this unavoidably dirty site is usually unnecessary and may be counterproductive in that overuse can alter the normal perineal microflora, encouraging colonization of the more resistant potential veneral disease producing bacteria *Klebsiella pneumoniae* and *Pseudomonas aeruginosa*.

ANALGESIA

The level of the pelvic brim is identified with a finger (Fig. 2.4). Lignocaine hydrochloride with adrenaline (Xylotox Veterinary; Willows Francis Veterinary) is infiltrated under the mucous membrane of both vulval lips, from just below the level of the pelvis to the upper commissure (Fig. 2.5).

SURGICAL TECHNIQUE

The perineum is washed again with water. Tissue forceps are used, at the muco-cutaneous junction, to raise the mucous membrane of one vulval lip. A strip of mucosa, approximately 4 mm wide, is removed from just below the level of the pelvic brim up to the upper commissure (Fig. 2.6). The procedure is repeated for the other vulval lip (Fig. 2.7). The denuded lips are checked for symmetry (Fig. 2.8) and are then sutured together, to just below the level of the pelvic brim, using monofilament or braided nylon, simple interrupted or continous interlocking suture patterns (Figs. 2.9 and 2.10). The latter pattern is preferred for mares who are operated upon for the first time and the former for repeat operations.

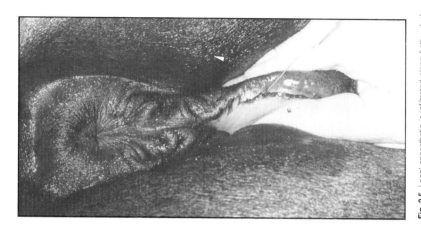

Fig. 2.5 Local anaesthetic is infiltrated along both vulval lips, at the mucocutaneous junction, from just below the level of the pelvis to the upper vulval commissure.

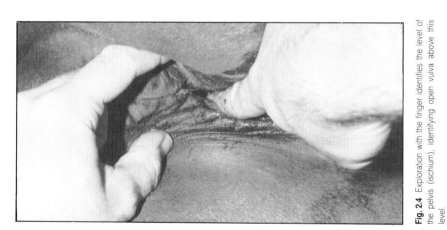

Fig. 2.4 Exploration with the finger identifies the level of the pelvis (ischium), identifying open vulva above this level.

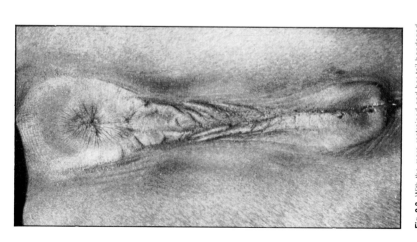

Fig. 2.3 With the mare restrained and her tail bandaged and held to one side, the perineum is prepared for surgery.

AFTERCARE

The completed suture line is washed with water and checked for uniform apposition of the vulval lips before sulphanilamide powder is applied (Fig. 2.11).

Daily intra-uterine antibiotic irrigations may be adminstered postoperatively, if indicated, through an indwelling uterine infuser (Arnolds), without disturbing the healing suture line (Figs. 2.12 and 2.13).

Attendants are advised to wash and apply sulphanilamide powder to the suture line daily for 7–10 days, at which time the sutures may be removed. When this operation is performed during the breeding season, removal of the sutures may result in wound breakdown at coitus. Sutures are thus often left in situ until the mare has been tested pregnant. Care must be

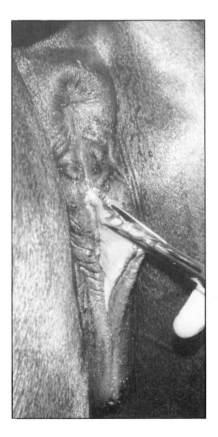

Fig. 2.6
Forceps (obscured behind the scissors) are placed at the mucocutaneous junction of one vulval lip, just below the level of the pelvis, and a strip of vulval mucosa approximately 4 mm wide, is removed with scissors.

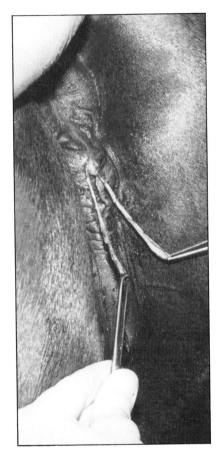

Fig. 2.7
Strips of mucosa are removed from both vulval lips, to the upper commissure.

taken to ensure that the stallion's penis is not injured by retained sutures.

MANAGEMENT

Reduced vulval aperture may provide managerial problems.

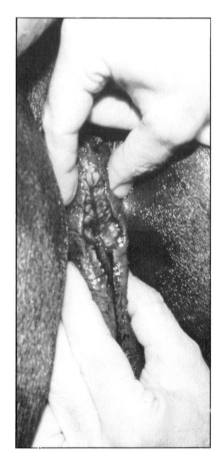

Fig. 2.8
The denuded vulval lips are checked for symmetry.

PARTURITION

An episiotomy must be performed prior to foaling otherwise major vulval or perineal damage may occur.

COITUS

An episiotomy must be performed on "tightly stitched" mares prior to natural coitus, otherwise injury to the stallion's penis or mare's vulva may occur. Episiotomy wounds must be repaired, as soon as possible, following foaling or coitus, to prevent a recurrence of pneumovagina, leading to acute

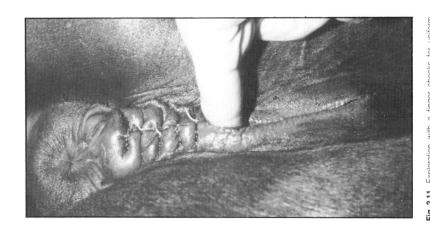

Fig. 2.11 Exploration with a finger checks for uniform apposition of the vulval lips and closure to just below the level of the pelvis.

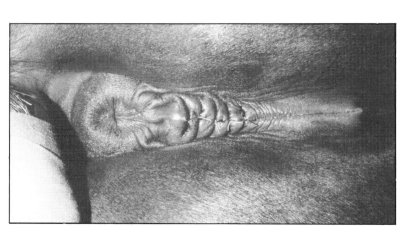

Fig. 2.10 The completed single interrupted suture line.

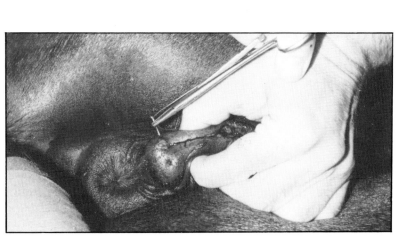

Fig. 2.9 The first suture is placed, to oppose the vulval lips.

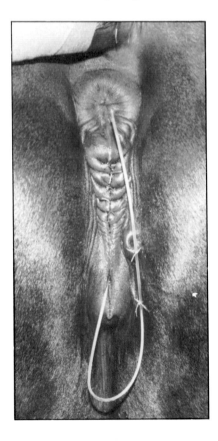

Fig. 2.12
An indwelling uterine infuser is placed in the uterine lumen and the distal end is stay-sutured to the vulvo-buttock junction.

endometritis and delayed uterine involution. Repeated episiotomy followed by closure leads to loss of vulval tissue, poor healing and, on occasions, major veterinary and managemental problems.

CAUSES OF UNSATISFACTORY RESULTS

SUTURE LINE BREAKDOWN

Postoperative infection is the most common cause of suture line breakdown. This is most commonly seen in post partum episiotomy wound repairs and in older mares which have been repeatedly repaired, especially during the spring "flush"

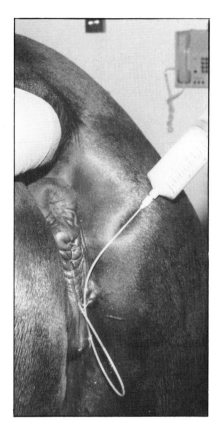

Fig. 2.13
Antibiotic solutions may be infused daily, via a 16
gauge hypodermic needle and syringe.

of grass when many mares show signs of diarrhoea. When
this happens, the sutures should be removed, local and
sometimes systemic antibiotic treatment applied and time
for healing and reepithelialization allowed before repair is
performed.

FISTULA FORMATION

A fistula may form in the suture line either following breakdown at one suture, where an excessive gap has been left
between adjacent sutures, or where inadequate mucosa has
been removed before closure. Sinus formation will result in
persistent pneumovagina and therefore must be identified at
suture removal and must be repaired.

CONCAVE VULVAL CONFORMATION

In mares with concave sloping vulvas, results are often poor even though the vulval lips have been sutured to the level of the clitoris.

UROVAGINA

The operation has no primary effect on urovagina.

ALTERNATIVE APPROACHES

In attempt to overcome the unwelcome sequelae associated with reduction of the vulval aperture, Pouret (1982) devised and described an alternative perineal reconstruction operation which corrects both pneumovagina and urovagina. This is, however, a more extensive surgical procedure which is used for selected cases. These may be mares who have a vulva which slopes, often in a concave manner (see above), to an extent that Caslick's operation cannot prevent pneumovagina or where urovagina is an additional problem.

REFERENCES AND FURTHER READING

Caslick, E.A. (1937). *Cornell Veterinarian* **27**, 178–187.

Pascoe, R. R. (1979). *Journal of Reproduction and Fertility* Supplement, **27**, 299–305.

Pickles, A. C. (1986). An assessment of the efficacy of perineal resection (Pouret 1982) for the surgical correction of pneumovagina in the mare. DESM Thesis, RCVS, London.

Pouret, E. J. M. (1982) *Equine Veterinary Journal* **14**, 249–250.

Ricketts, S. W. (1986). *Perineal Conformation Abnormalities. Current Therapy in Equine Medicine*, 2nd Edn (ed. N. E. Robinson) pp. 518–520, Eastbourne W. B. Saunders

Rossdale, P. D. & Ricketts, S. W. (1980). *Equine Studfarm Medicine*, 2nd Edn. London, Baillière Tindall.

Thornbury, R. S. (1975). *New Zealand Veterinary Journal* **23**, 277–280.

Walker, D. F. & Vaughan, J. T. (1980). *Bovine and Equine Urogenital Surgery*. Philadelphia, Lea & Febiger.

CHAPTER 3

A Surgical Approach to the Cryptorchid Horse

JOHN COX

INTRODUCTION

Any horse in which two testes are not visible and cannot be palpated in the scrotum must be suspected of being a cryptorchid.

DIAGNOSIS

Careful examination of the standing horse, perhaps after it has been tranquillized, may allow palpation of a testis which has been temporarily retracted under the influence of cold weather, fear or cold hands. Such testes are usually retained just above the scrotum and will usually be easily removed with the horse under general anaesthesia. If, however, the animal is left to mature further, the testis may descend to the scrotum.

Blood test

In animals which show male behaviour without any palpable testes, surgery should not be undertaken without the supporting evidence of a blood test. The age of the horse determines which test is carried out. In horses 3 years old and older, a single blood sample should be taken and submitted to a reputable laboratory which specializes in hormone estimations with a request for the measurement of conjugated oestrogens or conjugated oestrone sulphate. Donkeys, no matter what their age, and young horses should be subjected to the chorionic gonadotrophin stimulation test. In such animals it is necessary to take two blood samples, one before, and the other between 30 and 120 min after, the intravenous injection of 6000 iu of human chorionic gonadotrophin. The laboratory should be asked to measure testosterone which will indicate the presence of testes.

Palpation under anaesthesia

Deep palpation of the inguinal region may allow a testis which is retained high up to be palpated, but there are other structures which may be found there which can be difficult to distinguish from a testis without recourse to surgery. Failure to palpate a testis in the inguinal region does not mean that the horse does not have an inguinal testis.

It is rarely possible to palpate an abdominal testis per rectum. In animals in which the epididymal tail has descended, the ductus deferens can be felt passing through the vaginal ring but, as this can occur with the testis either within (so-called incomplete abdominal cryptorchidism) or outside the abdomen, the procedure is, in my opinion, of little value.

RESTRAINT FOR CRYPTORCHIDECTOMY

The horse should be restrained in dorsal recumbency under general anaesthesia (Fig. 3.1). Semi-lateral recumbency is unsuitable. Have it well enough anaesthetized to stay with hind legs relaxed. Prepare two areas for surgery. First, the scrotal and inguinal area, and second, if a testis cannot be positively palpated in the inguinal region, the suprapubic area – that is the area lateral to the opening of the sheath. Prepare this area on the side on which a testis is retained.

Starving the animal for 16 h before surgery empties the abdomen allowing abdominal testes to be found more easily.

INGUINAL EXPLORATION

Observation of the inguinal region may reveal a puckered scar on one side of a horse in dorsal recumbency (Fig. 3.2). This usually means that a testis has been removed from that side. A linear scar means very little.

Always explore the inguinal region surgically in order to find more positive evidence as to whether or not the horse has been castrated – don't rely solely upon palpation. Figure 3.3. shows where two incisions have been made in the scrotal

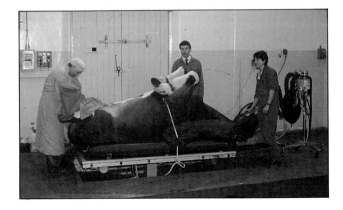

Fig. 3.1
Restraint for cryptorchidectomy.

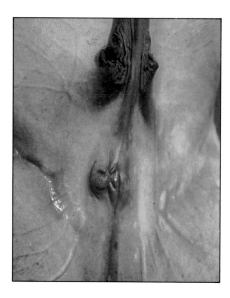

Fig. 3.2
The puckered scar on the right hand side of a horse in dorsal recumbency (the left as you look at it) usually means that a testis has been removed from that side.

area. The incisions are made here rather than over the inguinal canal for several reasons. First, it bleeds less here; second, the inguinal fat does not have to be displaced to get at the inguinal canal – you can burrow underneath it; third, the surgeon is following in reverse the path a testis should have taken to reach the scrotum, and surgical dissection along this line proceeds very easily. Once through the skin, use fingers to dissect towards the superficial inguinal ring (Fig. 3.4). This lies laterally and slightly cranially to an incision in the scrotum. Never use a scalpel to incise more than the skin. In this region there are large tributaries of the external pudendal vein. If one of these were nicked with a scalpel the surgical field would immediately be lost in a sea of blood.

Figure 3.5 shows the first view obtained of an inguinal testis. This is grasped with tissue forceps and pulled out through the incision to reveal the spermatic sac (Fig. 3.6) with its cremaster muscle and a testis inside it, and it can now be removed by any suitable procedure.

A stump of spermatic sac may be found in the inguinal area. It is about as thick as a thumb and reaches from the inguinal canal to the scrotum. The stump of spermatic sac is

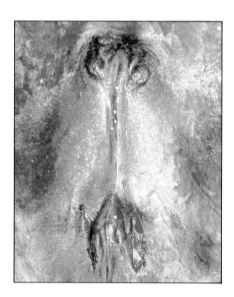

Fig. 3.3
Two incisions have been made in the scrotal area, prior to inguinal exploration. The opening of the sheath is at the top of the picture.

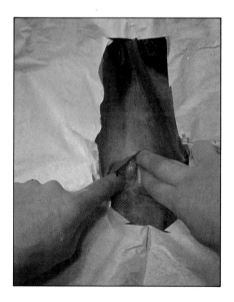

Fig. 3.4
Finger dissection towards the superficial inguinal ring.

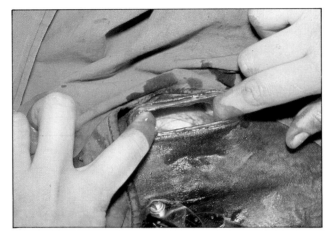

Fig. 3.5
The first view of an inguinal testis. The large area of glistening white is strongly suggestive of a spermatic sac containing a testis.

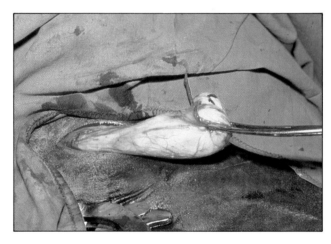

Fig. 3.6
Forceps extraction of the spermatic sac with cremaster muscle and testis inside it.

identified by the presence of a cremaster muscle round the outside of the white glistening tunic (Fig. 3.7). These stumps usually adhere to the scrotal scar.

The deferent duct and the remnants of testicular vessels can also be seen. Either remove about 5 cm of the stump or, as in Fig. 3.7, incise it where it is and look closely at the contents.

In order to be sure that this is the stump that remains after castration, it is necessary to identify:

Externally – the cremaster muscle and the white glistening sheet of vaginal tunic below it.

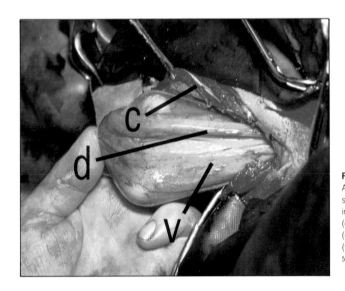

Fig. 3.7
A stump of spermatic
sac found in the
inguinal area
(c) cremaster muscle,
(d) deferent duct,
(v) remains of
testicular vessels.

Inside the vaginal tunic – Deferent duct (straw size, hard and white) and remnants of testicular vessels which looks like loose, fatty connective tissue. You may be able to identify cord-like remains of coiled testicular artery (this coiling can be confused with epididymis).

The remains of vessels are the most important thing to find – it is their presence that proves the animal has been castrated.

Figure 3.8 shows a spermatic sac, superfically very much like Figure 3.7 except that there are no adhesions between its distal end and the scrotum, and no scar in the scrotum. A cremaster muscle is also present. When this spermatic sac was incised the first thing to pop out was the tail of epididymis. This looks and feels like a coiled-up cord, something that is especially obvious if it is rolled between the fingers. When the spermatic sac has been incised for a longer distance, you may be able to see the coiled structure of the epididymis (Fig. 3.9). Going away from it on one side into the surgical wound is the deferent duct (identified by being straw sized, hard and white). On the other side is the body of the epididymis – identified in real life on very close inspection by its being composed of a very fine tightly coiled-up tube. This surgical finding in the inguinal area means that the case is one of incomplete abdominal cryptorchidism – the epididymal tail is descended but the testis is in the abdomen. By incising the

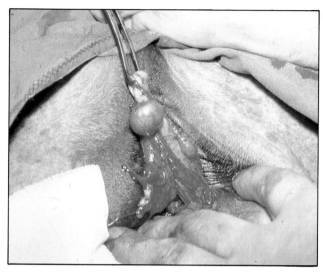

Fig. 3.8
A spermatic sac also showing the cremaster muscle.

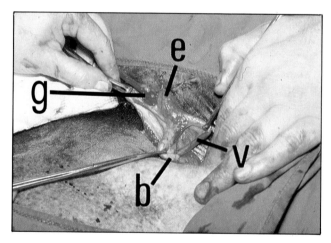

Fig. 3.9 Incision of the spermatic sac (b) body of the epididymis, (e) the epididymis, (g) the remains of the gubernaculum, (v) the deferent duct. The third pair of forceps in the upper left of the picture is holding the distal tip of the spermatic sac, attached to the tail of epididymis by a short cord, the remains of the gubernaculum.

spermatic sac to the level of the superficial inguinal ring, and applying traction to the body of the epididymis it is sometimes possible to deliver small testes out of the abdomen, as the body of the epididymis and the testis are connected to one another via the head of the epididymis. If traction does not deliver the testis, the structures should be removed using an emasculator and a laparotomy performed. Incomplete abdominal cryptorchidism is most likely to occur on the right side. In fact, a tail of epididymis will be found in about 50% of cases where the abdominally retained testis is on the right. Avoid the mistake of removing a tail of epididymis and calling it a misshapen testis by carefully identifying what is removed from a horse's inguinal region.

A spermatic sac emerging through the superficial inguinal ring at inguinal exploration is another possible finding (Fig. 3.10). When incised it was found to contain merely a fibrous cord. This fibrous cord is the remains of the gubernaculum which runs from epididymal tail to distal part of spermatic sac. In Figure 3.10 a testis complete with epididymis was found inside the abdomen. Traction on this gubernaculum may result in delivery of the testis and epididymis from the abdomen, but will not always do so – the testis attached to this gubernaculum weighed 365 g. If I find these structures in the inguinal region I proceed to a laparotomy to search for the abdominal testis.

Fat

One more inguinal finding remains to be mentioned – and that is fat. How to distinguish fat from spermatic sac is something that can only be learnt by looking and by feeling

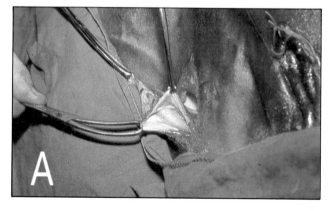

Fig. 3.10
A spermatic sac emerging through the superficial inguinal ring.

carefully. If necessary both left and right inguinal areas must be explored. The superficial inguinal ring itself should be clearly identified. With the horse on its back and with its legs relaxed as already described, the superficial inguinal ring is like a segment of a circle. The arc of this segment can be felt cranially as the tendinous edge of the abdominal tendon of the external oblique muscle, and the straight edge caudally as a very hard structure when the tendinous edge of the pelvic tendon of external oblique muscle is supported by the muscle and tendons of the medial thigh. The ring will usually admit two fingers. If it is clear that no spermatic sac passes through or lies just inside, then the testis must be in the abdomen.

SUPRA-PUBIC PARAMEDIAN LAPAROTOMY

MAKING THE INCISION

Techniques have been described which enter the abdomen through or close to the inguinal ring. These techniques, however, can be criticized on the grounds that they carry with them, even in experienced hands, the risk of intestinal prolapse and that it is bad surgery to make a hole in the abdominal wall that is difficult or impossible to suture. Moreover, the evidence is that animals operated upon in this way suffer considerable postoperative discomfort. In addition, these techniques have a high rate of technical failure in inexperienced hands as do those more recently described techniques which rely on identifying gubernaculum in spermatic sac deep in the inguinal region.

The technique of supra-pubic paramedian laparotomy has the merits that it is basically a conventional surgical approach to the abdomen, and it is, therefore, easier to understand than the rather mystical approach through the inguinal ring, and (lastly but not least), experience with over 300 laparotomies for retained testes at the Liverpool veterinary school has shown that the technique is free of major complications.

The area for laparotomy is that immediately lateral to the opening of the sheath (Fig. 3.11) so the horse need not be moved from its position of dorsal recumbency. The surgeon, therefore, should move to a position alongside the horse on the side of retention.

The exact location of the incision varies slightly with the horse. Try to avoid any large skin vessels, although more problems of haemorrhage are likely to be encountered in incising the fat which underlies the skin than in the skin itself. Make the incision long enough to put a hand in. The fat is the next layer to be cut through. Once the skin and subcutaneous fat have been cut through, the yellow abdominal tunic is exposed (Fig. 3.12). This must be incised along the length of the incision and the incision must go through the tendons of external and internal oblique muscles which are usually adherent to the dorsal surface of the yellow abdominal tunic.

The result of the incision through the tunic is to expose the underlying straight abdominal muscle whose fibres run parallel to the line of incision and which can, therefore, be split along the line of its fibres (Fig. 3.13).

This procedure usually gives a blood-free view of the tendon of the transverse muscle, the fibres of which run at right angles to the line of the incision. There is a choice. If your hand is small puncture the transverse tendon with a closed pair of blunt scissors and push a finger and then a hand into the abdomen so splitting the tendon along its fibres. This gives a grid iron approach to the abdominal cavity which is easy to repair. It does, however, make a rather small hole.

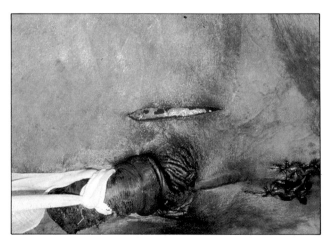

Fig. 3.11
Skin incision for
paramedian
laparotomy on the left
side of the horse.

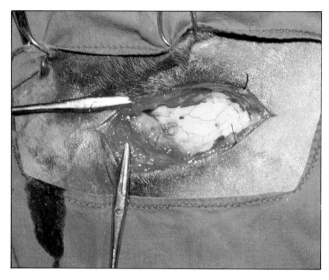

Fig. 3.12
Exposure of the
yellow abdominal
tunic, having cut
through the skin and
subcutaneous fat.

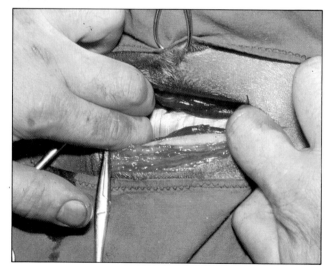

Fig. 3.13
Splitting of straight
abdominal muscle
fibres.

Those with large muscular fists will find it better to incise
the tendon along the line of the skin incision. Underlying the
transverse tendon and adherent to it is the peritoneum, but
as the peritoneum of the horse is very fine and delicate,

incising the tendon usually means gaining direct access through the peritoneal cavity. Care should, therefore, be taken when making this incision. Occasionally in very fat ponies a layer of fat lies between the transverse tendon and peritoneum. Variable amounts of fluid escape from the peritoneal cavity when it is entered, but this is usually of no concern.

LOCATING AND REMOVING THE TESTIS

What clues do we have as to where the testis is, for after all the abdominal cavity is a very large cavity to search? In the pig shown in Figure 3.14 the epididymal tail and testis are closely attached to the deep (or internal) inguinal ring through which the vaginal process has passed. The first place to look for an abdominal testis is therefore here, just inside the deep inguinal ring. This lies just caudal to the previously described incision in the abdominal wall and through which a hand has been put to find the testis. The hand must be kept close to

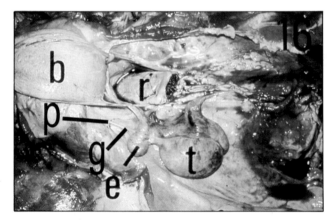

Fig. 3.14 Post mortem dissection of a cryptorchid pig. The pig's head is to the right and most of the body wall has been cut away, together with the intestines. The bladder (b) has been picked up and reflected over the pelvis to expose the transected rectum (r) in which black faeces can be seen. Below this in the picture lie the testis (t) and the epididymal tail (e). The epididymal body can be seen above the testis running behind the peritoneal fold which suspended the testis from the dorsal body wall and a ligament can be clearly seen running from testis to epididymal tail. This ligament continues beyond the tail of the epididymis as a thinner strand (g) and can be seen to enter a pouch of peritoneum (p). This pouch is the vaginal process which has pushed through the deep inguinal ring and the ligament that we've just described is part of the gubernaculum. In fact this would be the abdominal view of the structures seen in the inguinal relgion in Fig. 3.10.

the abdominal wall to avoid getting tangled up with intestine and usually needs inserting only up to the wrist at this stage. The testis itself is usually both small and flabby, not at all like a scrotal testis. So the first point that helps locate an abdominal testis is the fact that most such testes lie close to the deep inguinal ring.

Running from the epididymal tail to the neck of the bladder is the left deferent duct (on the pig's right side you can see the right deferent duct entering a vaginal process – on that side the testis was in the scrotum). The position of the deferent duct on the dorsal surface of the neck of the bladder is fixed anatomically. By finding it by palpation and then following back along the duct to the tail of the epididymis and then along the body to the head of the epididymis, the testis can usually be found. This technique of following the deferent duct and epididymis from the dorsal surface of the neck of the bladder to the testis is very useful if the testis doesn't lie close to the deep inguinal ring. A large proportion of abdominal testes lie close to the neck of the bladder anyway so the testis may be found while trying to locate the deferent duct. In such a case, the arm may need to be inserted to mid forearm. Throughout abdominal explorations the hand should be kept close to the body wall – equine intestine is sticky and it can be difficult to disengage a hand from a mass of small intestine.

Sometimes, unfortunately, the testis is not located by either of these means and a blind search of the caudal abdomen has to be made. In such a case, the most important thing to remember is that the abdominal testis is usually flabby and small and therefore feels very different from a scrotal testis. Occasionally, however, you will meet the grossly distorted teratomatous or cystic testis. The most useful thing that can be said in addition, is that the epididymal tail has a characteristic feel and that you can learn this sensation by practising on normal scrotal testes that you remove. Feel for the tubules within the relatively thin capsule and roll them gently between your fingers. If the epididymal tail is found within the abdomen this leads to the testis.

Assuming you've found the testis, bring it out through the surgical incision (Fig. 3.15). Sometimes it comes out easily, but not always. Place a good emasculator (e.g. a Serra) round the blood vessels – our experience is that ligatures are not then necessary.

Don't worry about removing all the epididymis if it won't come out through the incision – there is no evidence that it produces androgens and a bit has often been left behind without any consequences. We always make sure we've removed all the testis – it's that that produces testosterone.

Once the testis is removed, the incision is then closed. Figure 3.16 shows a representation of the first suture. When tied, this suture closes the grid-iron incision in its centre. Next suture the yellow abdominal tunic and adherent tendons

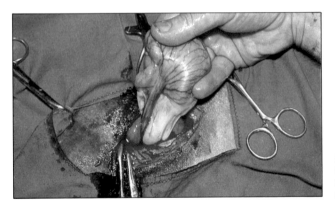

Fig. 3.15 Extraction of the testis through a surgical incision.

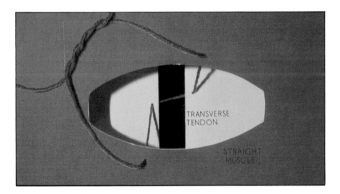

Fig. 3.16 Diagrammatic representation of the first suture, placed to close the tears in the transverse tendon and the straight abdominal muscle. This is done by taking the suture down through the straight muscle on the medial side (the upper part of the picture), down through the transverse tendon on the cranial side (the right side of the picture), up through the transverse tendon on the cranial side (the right side of the picture), up through the transverse tendon on the caudal left side and up through the straight abdominal muscle on the lateral (lower) side.

with horizontal mattress sutures, the fat with a continuous suture and finally the skin with horizontal mattress sutures.

Always make sure that gut is not trapped in this suture – this is also made less likely by the animal starving for 16 h before surgery. If desired, one interrupted suture in the straight abdominal muscle may be put on each side of this one. (If the transverse tendon had to be cut along the line of the skin incision it will be necessary to place several interrupted sutures through the tendon and muscle together, again making sure intestine isn't trapped in the sutures.)

COMPLICATIONS

(1)   One horse which developed severe colic several days after the operation was found to have intestine trapped in the suture line. It hadn't been starved properly.

(2)   Before synthetic absorbable suture materials became available, a number of horses developed marked oedema around the laparotomy wound, sometimes so extensive as to cause wound breakdown. Now that we use synthetic absorbable sutures, the amount of oedema which develops seems to be more related to the trauma necessary to get a hand into and a large testis out of the abdomen.

(3)   Occasionally, a horse develps mild colic a few hours after surgery. As the same thing happens in other anaesthetized horses the abdomens of which haven't been entered, this isn't always related to handling intestine. A single injection of pethidine hydrochloride is usually effective.

(4)   Most horses look bright and alert the day after surgery, but occasionally a horse will look miserable. In such a case we give three extra daily injections of crystalline penicillin and, again, the animal responds quickly – perhaps these horses have mild peritonitis.

FURTHER READING

The technique of supra-pubic paramedian laparatomy was first described by Marcel in 1838, but fell into disuse until rediscovered by Professor J.G. Wright in 1955 and described by him in *The Veterinary Record* **72**, 57–60.

Further details of the technique and an account of the phenomenon of cryptorchidism in the horse will be found in *Surgery of the Reproductive Tract in Large Animals* by J. E. Cox. Liverpool University Press.

CHAPTER 4

Air Hygiene and Equine Respiratory Disease

A. CLARKE

INTRODUCTION

The importance of environmental factors on the welfare of the horse has long been appreciated. Percivall (1853) highlighted this point by introducing his treatise on respiratory disease of the horse as follows:

"No general fact appears better established in hippopathology than the one evidencing that disease is the penalty that nature has attached to the domestication of the horse."

Chronic pulmonary disease (CPD) is one such affliction. Clinically, CPD is associated with varying degres of dyspnoea and double expiratory effort. In its initial stages, however, the disease may pass undetected until the horse undertakes heavy exertion, as in racing.

This chapter examines those aspects of the air hygiene and the aerobiology of stables as they relate to the pathophysiology and management of CPD in all of its manifestations. Simple guidelines for, and practical approaches to the assessment of the air hygiene of stables are described.

AETIOLOGY

Factors known to be associated with clinically overt cases of CPD include mouldy feeds and beddings, poorly ventilated stables and previous viral and bacterial infections. Subclinical lower airway inflammatory disease has been associated with "poor performance" of thoroughbreds. This condition is known as Lower Respiratory Tract Inflammation (LRTI). Diagnosis of this condition is based on the presence of increased mocopus and inflammatory cells (neutrophils) revealed by endoscopic examination and tracheal washings. Bacterial and viral respiratory tract infections and large airborne challenges of respirable dust have been individually implicated as having aetiological roles in LRTI, and together they appear to act synergistically. (In much the same way, children are more prone to asthma after respiratory tract infections.) Airway hyperactivity is now a well-documented feature of respiratory tract disease in horses and horses so affected have a lowered tolerance to inhaled particles and noxious gases of all kinds.

AIRBORNE CONTAMINANTS OF STABLES

Stabled horses are exposed to a myriad of airborne contaminants. These include fungal and actinomycete spore clouds, bacterial and viral aerosols, noxious gases such as ammonia, plant material, dust mites and their metabolites. These contaminants may be pathogenic in a number of ways. They may cause infection, be allergenic, behave as primary irritants or simply "clog" the respiratory defence mechanism, so increasing the system's susceptibility to other pathogens.

The sources of, and clearance mechanisms for the airborne contaminants of stables are presented in Fig. 4.1. Respirable challenges of mould spores will depend on the degree of contamination of feed and bedding. Airborne mould spores and noxious gases are cleared mainly by ventilation. The short survival time of many viruses and bacteria in air ensures that much of their infectious potential is lost before they are removed by ventilation. Nevertheless, they may still be harmful simply because of their potential "clogging" effects on the respiratory tract defence mechanisms.

Infectious respiratory disease may be transmitted by a number of routes other than aerosol dispersion. These include direct contact, e.g. nose-to-nose, indirect contact via tack or handlers, or direct droplet transmission, e.g. from an infected horse coughing directly on to a susceptible horse. This combination of transmission modalities and the wide range of environmental conditions which favour the survival of infectious pathogens (e.g. equine herpesvirus-1 favours low humidity and equine rhinovirus-1 high humidity) ensures that environmental management cannot really alter the spread of highly contagious infectious agents through a fully susceptible population of horses.

The most promising means of controlling infectious respiratory disease is by vaccination, although further research is necessary to increase both efficacy and duration of effect.

$$R = C(q_v + q_s + q_a + q_d + q_g)$$

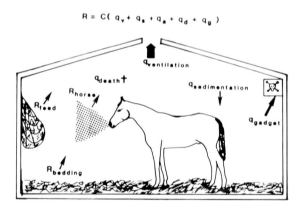

Fig. 4.1 Balance of airborne contaminants. The airborne concentration (C) of a pathogen is proportional to the rate of its release (R) into and rate of its clearance (q) from the air. Fungal spores may be released from feed and bedding (R feed and bedding), viruses and bacteria from the horse itself (R horse) and noxious gases from bedding. Clearance may be via direct removal of the pathogen from the air (primarily involving ventilation q_v) or removal of its pathogenic potential while airborne (death of infectious agent q_d). Less significant clearance mechanisms include (i) sedimentation (q_s–very slow for small particles), (ii) breathing of the horse (q_a) and (iii) gadgetry (q_g e.g. air filters). These gadgets are usually inefficient for the size of building in which they are located and poorly maintained. Courtesy of *Equine Veterinary Journal* (Clarke 1987a).

AIR HYGIENE MANAGEMENT

Air hygiene management based on minimizing exposure to airborne pollutants will decrease the recovery time following an infectious disease, and lower the incidence of lifelong complications following a short-term infection.

The safe levels or threshold limiting values for airborne contaminants in relation to diseases of the respiratory tract of the horse are unknown. Indeed, they can vary, a horse with a respiratory tract infection being likely to have a lower tolerance to inhaled contaminants than before the infection. As the degree of respiratory embarrassment to most of these pollutants is likely to be dependent on the level of challenge, such challenges should be minimized at all times. There are two approaches to reduce the concentrations of airborne pollutants in stables:

(1)   Increase clearance rates (primarily via ventilation)
(2)   Reduce release rates (by modifying source materials)

The importance of using both these approaches is illustrated in Fig. 4.2. The use of clean source materials will minimize challenges of airborne mould spores. However, ignoring ventilation can lead to fungal growth in bedding materials, problems with condensation and can promote the spread of infectious diseases. Equally, horses exposed to contaminated feeds and bedding may inhale significant levels of particles even though a recording instrument on a table in the middle of the box may show apparently low levels. A susceptible horse eating contaminated hay in the ultimate of natural ventilation, i.e. an open field, will cough!

VENTILATION OF BUILDINGS

The efficiency of ventilation will be most severely tested in still air conditions. Probable ventilation rates may be calculated from the dimensions of the building, its inlets and outlets and the sensible heat loss from horses (approximated at 6.3 W/kg) (Table 4.1.) Minimal ventilation rates can be pre-

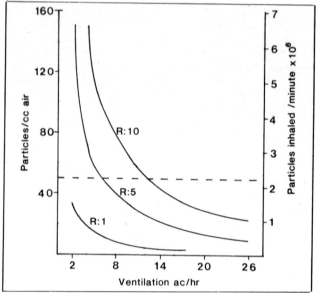

Fig. 4.2 The effect of ventilation in air changes per hour (ac/hour) on the numbers of respirable particles per cc of air at three relase rates of particles (n/cc air per min). Assumes tidal volume of 3 and 15 breaths/min.
R = 1 corresponds to conditions which exist when bedding and fodder are almost entirely free of contamination. Such a situation exists when the bedding is clean wood shavings (or very clean paper) and the hay is soaked before feeding.
R = 5 corresponds to conditions existing, e.g. when good quality straw is used for bedding and changed daily.
R = 10 corresponds to conditions where bedding or fodder are significantly contaminated with fungal spores.
These graphs are based on steady state levels at quiet periods in daytime and do not allow for increased levels of dust at mucking-out. If the interrupted line at 50 particles per cc or 2.3 m × 10⁶ particles inhaled per minute is taken as a threshold limiting value at low release rates, i.e. very clean bedding and food, this value is not exceeded until ventilation rates are 1 ac/h. At higher release rates ventilation must be increased. However, the horse may still inhale high levels of dust as it sniffs at a contaminated feed or bedding.

dicted, using a computer analysis of these parameters. However, such analyses take no account of the distributions of openings or mixing of air within a building. It must also be remembered that still air conditions are rarely maintained for long. The design of new stables and improvement of existing stables should be related to the natural landscape and prevailing weather conditions, especially wind direction and sun.

Actual ventilation rates of buildings may be assessed with either an inert tracer gas such as sulphur hexafluoride and an autoanalyser, or the clearance of smoke clouds using an airborne particle counter such as the Rion KC01A (Hawksley; West Sussex).

These techniques are efficient but relatively expensive and beyond economical justification for the majority of practices.

Table 4.1 The three natural forces of ventilation. Building design and the positioning of inlet and outlets should maximize the effects of these three forces.

Stack effect – warm air rises from the horses acting as a driving force for ventilation.
Aspirations – wind blowing across the top of a building will draw air from the building with proper outlets.
Perflation – air blowing from side to side and end to end provides ventilation.

Specialist services are available to carry out such work, investigating existing stables and liaising with architects and owners on new projects to ensure optimum environmental conditions are provided for the stabled horse (Equigiene; Wrington, Avon). A more economical and practical approach is to measure air movement patterns within a building using smoke tubes or smoke bombs. These tubes also give an indication of the functional state of vents and ducting, providing visual and often graphic on-the-spot demonstrations.

Draughts

Another useful and relatively inexpensive device is a wind speed anemometer. This may be used to assess air movement inside and outside buildings and for draught detection. Draughts are basically too much ventilation in the wrong place causing enhanced heat loss and chilling in cold weather. They are especially of significance for the neonate. A draught has arbitrarily been defined as a wind speed of greater than 0.4 m/s at animal height. The arbitrary nature of this definition can be appreciated by bearing in mind that the chilling effect of a wind blowing on a neonate is considerably more than the same "draught" blowing on to an adult horse with a rug. Returning to the neonate, minimization of draughts may not be enough to avoid hypothermia, especially if the foal is immature or ill. A dry, deep bedding avoiding direct contact with concrete is essential. New highly efficient insulating materials used as rugs e.g. Flectalon (Bulwark Industrial Estate,

Chepstow) are also very useful. Draughts may be prevented with the correct design and positioning of inlets and use of baffling.

Recommendations for the ventilation of animal houses are often given in terms of volumetric air movement, e.g. per m^3 of air per hour. The ventilation rate will be dependent on the air space per horse so the critical consideration must be for air changes per hour (ac/h). Big American-type barns are more difficult to ventilate than individual boxes. This is due to:

(a)   The large amounts of air which need to be moved to maintain adequate ac/hour
(b)   Poor mixing of air within the barn
(c)   Warm air rising from the horses may cool before it reaches outlets.

Barns provide more economical accommodation and easier working conditions for staff than individual boxes. Series of smaller barns are preferable to individual larger barns since they allow the benefits of this style of accommodation and more efficient ventilation through natural forces. Big barns can be successfully ventilated, however, many basic faults are often incorporated into their design. These include inadequate and poorly distributed ventilation, long low buildings, enclosed boxes within barns, poor lighting and feed and bedding storage in shared air spaces with the horses.

Openings

The distribution of openings within the buildings is as critical as the size of the openings. Open top doors in a loose-box provide adequate inlet areas and with a suitably sized opening in the back wall of a box with a monopitch roof, ventilation should be adequate until the top door is closed. Three openings are preferable for such boxes; the top door, outlet in back wall, and inlet in front wall to ensure adequate ventilation when the door is closed.

Boxes which have peaked roofs should ideally have a fourth opening in the form of a capped chimney. Large barns require an even greater distribution of opening to ensure adequate mixing of air and thorough ventilation of all individual boxes under one roof. This is most easily achieved by the use of Yorkshire boarding rather than a small number of individual openings, and a capped ridge along the roof (Fig. 4.3).

The recommendations in Table 4.2 provide useful guidelines for the assessment of stabling. However, in designing new stables or improving existing buildings, calculations for the individual structures are necessary. Landscape and prevailing weather conditions must be taken into account, especially for the distribution and design of inlets and outlets.

The effects of prevailing winds and the entry of rain and

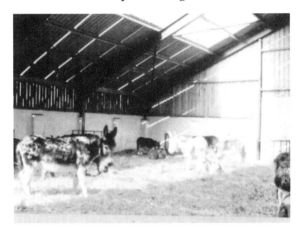

Fig. 4.3
Extensive use of Yorkshire boarding, a breathing roof and a clear perspex skylight, are features of this barn which make full use of natural resources for ventilation.

Table 4.2 Theoretical guidelines for inlet and outlet areas to provide four air changes per hour.

	Outlet	Inlet
Uninsulated loosebox (50 m^3 air space per horse)	0.20	0.35
Insulated loosebox (50 m^3 air space per horse)	0.15	0.30
Uninsulated barn (85 m^3 air space per horse)	0.25	0.50
Insulated barn (85 m^3 air space per horse)	0.20	0.40

The air space allowances are very generous. These guidelines are therefore adequate for most types of horse housing (After Webster *et al.* 1987).

snow may be reduced with Netlon (Windbreak), Yorkshire boarding, adjustable space boarding or shielded vents. Yorkshire boarding and Netlon may be used extensively in big barns to aid the maintenance of adequate ventilation. Netlon also provides excellent temporary wind-breaks.

Capped chimneys and ridges or elevated roof lights provide outlets for rising warm air and for the ventilatory effects of aspiration. Skylights or clear perspex sheeting allow extra light into a stable and if elevated with an overhang to the rest of the roof, they will allow natural ventilation without access to rain and snow. Upturned corrugated sheeting with a 15 mm spacing between sheets may be used to create a venturi slot between sheets for extractor ventilation. This is the so called "breathing roof". The small amount of rain which may enter through the slots is usually more than compensated for with the decreases in condensation because of improved ventilation.

New boxes should be positioned or alterations carried out to old boxes so as to make full use of natural resources. Boxes facing just east of south in England will get the benefit of morning sun, especially in winter. An overhang over the front of the boxes will help to protect the horses from rain and snow and give a covered area for staff. Rows of boxes may also be staggered down a slope or slight hill to get full advantage of morning sun to all boxes.

Another natural resource often overlooked is access to fresh air through an open door or window. Closing the top door of most conventionally-designed boxes in still air conditions inhibits ventilation. Opening the big end doors in barns or placing vents in them enhances ventilation. Cleaning blocked vents and ducts and opening windows apparently closed since their construction in Victorian days, may be all that is needed with older stabling. An open top door or window in a box with a V bar fitted to stop weaving, allows ready access to fresh air. The introduction of these V bars does not keep horses away from their feed and probably allays some of the boredom associated with being stabled up to 22 h per day. Doors or adjustable windows on the out-facing walls of barns improve ventilation as well as allowing access to fresh air.

Mechanical ventilation

In buildings which are excessively wide or long, or under conditions of climatic extremes, mechanical ventilation may be beneficial. These systems should be associated with the best use of natural flow forces. Inlets should be well distributed to aid thorough mixing of air. In very large barns overhead fans may minimize "stagnation" in the central rows of boxes.

Air filters provide an effective form of ventilation depending on their volumetric capacity and filter efficiency. However, there is little benefit in raising ventilation above the six to eight air changes per hour which is normally achievable with natural ventilation. Where such levels cannot be achieved either because of design or management constraints, building size and distribution of units should be fully assessed. Small units designed primarily for pubs and clubs are usually not appropriate for stables.

No beneficial effects of ionizers on dust level in stables have been observed. Negative ions may have some intrinsic (yet to be proven) benefit to the equine respiratory system. Ionizers and air filters may be of greater use in intensive livestock housing where natural ventilation is not possible or appropriate with, for example, the constraints on temperature control. However, they seem unlikely to bestow any benefit to the horse in a well-ventilated stable. Mechanical equipment may break down and the regular cleaning and maintenance required, though initially enthusiastically carried out, is usually soon neglected. "Investment" in gadgetry may better be placed in building modifications and use of alternative feed and bedding materials.

It must be remembered, however, that access to unlimited fresh air will be of little value to the horse with its nose held close to mouldy hay or sniffing at mouldy bedding.

Air hygiene assessment

In stables, the primary sources of respiratory dusts are mouldy hays and straws and growth *in situ* of fungi on bedding materials of plant origin such as wood shavings and diced newspaper. Some fungal growth may occur on stable walls as a result of condensation (Fig. 4.4) or more commonly, seepage of water through walls because of damaged drainage (Fig. 4.5).

Qualitative and quantitative descriptions of these substrates as sources of spores per unit of weight and the effects on the air hygiene of stables are presented in Tables 4.3 and 4.4. These analyses involve the use of culture procedures using various combinations of media and incubation temperatures, multistage impactor samplers and particle counters. Expensive equipment and staff beyond the reach of small practice laboratories are required. However, a quick semi-quantitative assessment for the degree of mould contamination of the various source materials may be carried out in practice. This involves the use of a hand held single-stage personal air sampler (Equigiene; Wrington, Avon). A biscuit of hay or straw is agitated and the sampler held in the dust cloud about 30 cm from the hay for 3 s.

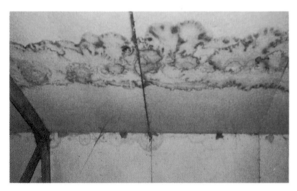

Fig. 4.4
Pattern staining on roof insulation is a typical sign of condensation problems and poor ventilation.

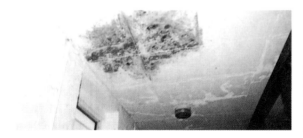

Fig. 4.5
Moulds or algae growing on the roof or walls are associated with a leaking roof, damaged drain pipes or condensation.

Samples of shavings, oats, etc. may be placed in a large paper bag and shaken before sampling in the bag. The sampler may also be run in the stable and above bedding material to check for moulding *in situ*. Once a sample is collected it is categorized according to the presence of plant material and mould spores. The sampler may be run for longer periods and by counting strips of known width across the stage the total number of particles from a set volume of air (the sampler runs at 10 l/min) may be calculated and identified.

HAYS

Some degree of fungal contamination is present in all hays (Fig. 4.6). Heated hays are very dusty and the composition of the dust is primarily thermophilic fungi and actinomycetes.

The most critical factor in determining the microbial development in hay is the water content at baling. Hay that is baled with 15–20 % water content heats little. It is virtually dust free with some plant debris or pollen grains (Fig. 4.7). There may be small numbers of spores but they will primarily be the normal constituents of the so-called "field fungi" or "fine weather air spora".

Baling hay at 20–30 % may lead to temperatures of 35–45°C with moderate amounts of mould contamination which may include large numbers of allergens and infectious pathogens (e.g. *Scopulariopsis brevicaulis* and *Aspergillus fumigatus*). Baling at 35–50 % water content leads to spontaneous heating of up to 50–60°C. It is under these conditions that the worst contamination of hay and straw occurs, with respirable challenges of up to 10^{10} fungal and actinomycete propagules per breath as the horse eats mouldy hay from a hay net (Fig. 4.8).

The dust mite (Fig. 4.9) adds a further complicating factor. It is dependent on fungal spores for food. The spores are replaced with clumps of semi-digested spores in the form of faecal pellets. The mites may be found in hay stored for many months or they may disappear much earlier. If the mites disappear, the only evidence will be faecal pellets and the occasional exoskeleton. A hay sample which has large amounts of mites or their faecal pellets, even without large numbers of

Table 4.3 Comparisons of particulate release rates and fungal contamination of various bedding materials, hay and silages.

	Beddings						Hay and silages			
	Equi-bed	Fen-pol	Diced news-paper	Shavings (range)	Straw (range)	Tissue	Rye (range)	Lucerne (range)	Horse-hage	Silage
Particles per mg*	19	4	78	148 873	1490 28100	53	980 65200	840 39270	44	19
Proportion of particles (%)**										
Fungal and actinomycete particles	ng	ng	ng	5 96	90 100	ng	30 99	55 90	5	5
Plant material	ng	ng	ng	95 4	8 trace	ng	70 ng	45 ng	95	95
Other	100	100	100	ng ng	2 trace	100	ng 1	ng 1	ng	ng
Culture analysis***	—	—	—	MF+ MF++ TF TA+	MF++ MF+ "field fungi" -TF+++ TA+ TCA++	—	MF+ TA "field fungi" -TCA+++ MF+ TF+++ TCA+++	MF MF TF+++ TA+ TCA+++	—	—

*Assessed using laser based aerodynamic particle sizer **Assessed using May Impactor ***Assessed using Andersen sampler
MF, Mesophilif fungi (25°C); TA, Thermotolerant actinomycete (38°C); TF, Thermotolerant fungi (38°C); TCA, Thermophilic actinomycete (55°C).
Equibed – Melcourt Industries, Tetbury, Gloucestershire (absorbent synthetic bedding).
Fenpol – Raymond Barnes Bloodstock, Newmarket (non-absorbent synthetic bedding).
Diced newspaper – Shredabed, Exeter.
Tissue bedding – F. H. Lee, Bolton, Greater Manchester.
ng, negligible.

Table 4.4 Comparison of different beddings and their management (After Clarke 1987b).

	Equibed*	Shavings*	Shavings** (dirty)	Shavings (deep litter)	Straw*	Paper*	Paper (deep litter)
Particles/cm³ air***	1-5	6-104	603	400-1223	167-724	25-100	62-1296
Description of mould contamination	Negligible	Negligible	Primary mould spores	Primary mould spores very heavy	Primary mould spores heavy-very heavy	Moderate	Very heavy

Particle counts are increases in numbers per cm³ of stable air which result from bedding down.
* Daily mucking out.
** Daily mucking out in poorly ventilated heavily insulated (hot and humid) barn.
*** Increases at mucking out, i.e., time of maximum dust release from bedding using RION KCOIA 5-channel particle counter.
In deep litter management systems and under warm humid climatic conditions fungal contamination of bedding may occur.

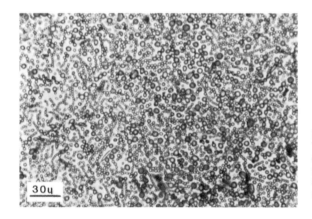

Fig. 4.6
Typical photomicrograph of contaminated hay, straw or plant-based bedding. There are large numbers of small respirable fungal spores.

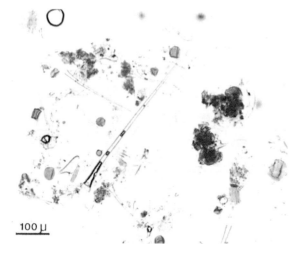

Fig. 4.7
A clean hay sample with minimal fungal contamination. a, Fragments of plant tissue; b, Plant hairs; c, Pollen grains. Courtesy of *Equine Veterinary Journal*, Clarke and Madelin (1987).

spores, must be considered as poor quality. The viability of spores is not essential to their allergenicity and dust mites are allergenic in their own right as well as releasing allergens from the ingested spores.

Although the health risks of mouldy hay are apparently well appreciated within the equine fraternity, heavily contaminated hays are regularly found at all levels of the horse world from the hay net at the pony club event to the manger of the most expensive thoroughbreds. Exorbitant prices (up to £10 per bale) are paid for imported hays on the false assumption that

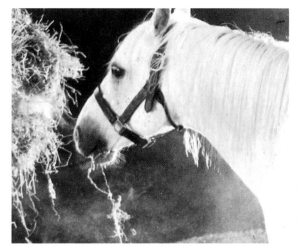

Fig. 4.8
Counts of up to 4000
respirable fungal spores per
cc of air may be recorded
around a hay net or feeder
with mouldy hay. At a 2·5 l
tidal volume this equates to
10^7 fungal spores per breath.

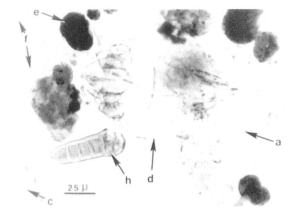

Fig. 4.9
Dust mite (d) present in dust
collected from mouldy hay; e,
Mite excreta; c, Pollen grain;
a, Plant material; f, Small
respirable fungal spore; h,
helminthosporium spore.
Courtesy of *Equine Veterinary
Journal*, Clarke and Madelin
(1987).

quality is dependent on price alone. However, such hays, especially the lucernes, can be heavily contaminated. The price premiums paid for these hays seems unjustified on both air hygiene and nutritional grounds, although there is apparent increased palatability associated with lucerne and clover hays.

Even though the pre-baling addition of preservatives such as propionic acid may significantly decrease the total spore burden of hay baled at high moisture content, numbers and species of moulds capable of producing hypersensitive airway diseases still develop.

Significant fungal contamination can also occur with barn-dried hay. Traditional barn-dried hay is baled within a few days of cutting and is stored with air vents through the stack. As the most serious moulding occurs within the first few days after baling, hay which is baled with a high moisture content may still become heavily moulded. More recently, two approaches have been taken to overcome this problem. Hay-Tek (Greens of Sohan) is producing suitable mixtures of ryegrass which are cut and wilted, then placed loose in large drying kilns. The hay is low-temperature dried by forcing air through the crop. It is baled with a low moisture content and heavy moulding is therefore avoided. The alternative approach involves the use of large, high-temperature driers which process large quantities of grass. Special care must be taken in the curing process to avoid damage to protein. This is achieved with a suitable initial wilting and drying phase in the field.

Soaking hay

Soaking of hay reduces the respirable challenge to the horse. The duration of soaking is not as important as thorough wetting. A quick dip into a bucket of water or a sprinkle from a watering can is not sufficient. A 10 min soak is sufficient as long as the hay is completely wetted. Likewise, sitting a bale in water for 12 h without cutting the strings may not allow access of water to the centre of the bale. The simplest management procedure is to soak hay on a 12-hour basis, i.e. the evening's hay is immersed in water in the morning. While soaking of hay prevents the airborne release and inhalation of spores, the spores are still ingested. Depending on the species that are present, problems with mycotoxins and infections may occur. Heavily-moulded hay has also undergone biochemical changes which can alter its nutritional status. Damped, contaminated hay which drops to the floor may "seed" a biological bedding with fungi.

An alternative to soaking hay is to use a mechanical cleaner. This equipment agitates hay while vacuuming the airborne spores away ("Dust Cure", Sedgemoor Developments; Bridgwater, Somerset).

Silages and haylage offer possible cleaner alternatives to

hays. They must be packed airtight and used within a few days of opening. Botulism in horses has been associated with the feeding of big bale silage. The risk of botulism from big bale silage may be minimized by using only airtight bags and avoiding bales which have a pH less than 5, which give off the smell of ammonia when opened or which contain dirt. Opened bags of silage will mould rapidly unless preservatives have been used and should be fed within 3 days of opening.

BEDDINGS

The other major source of fungal spores is bedding. Straw has been the traditional bedding. Straw that has been baled damp has a very similar microflora to a heated hay and is just as dangerous. However, the fungi associated with "clean" straw (Fig. 4.10) are usually of the large spore type. Paper beddings, peat moss and woodshavings are usually practically free of fungi and actinomycetes when fresh. However, they may cause problems in deep litter management systems or if they heat up in warm, poorly ventilated stables. The non-biological beddings are very clean, thermally efficient and do not provide a base medium for fungal growth. Tissue bedding impregnated with disinfectant also provides a good, clean bedding when fresh and inhibits growth of microbes *in situ*. Concern over

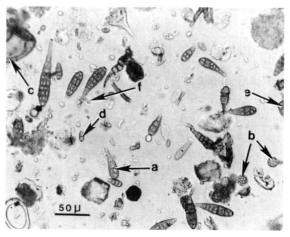

Fig. 4.10
A typical "clean" non-heated straw sample with "fine weather air spora". a, Alternaria spore; b, Rust spore; c, Pollen grain; d, Cladosporium spore; e, Damaged helminthosporium spore; f, Aspergillus/penicillium spores. Courtesy of *Equine Veterinary Journal*, Clarke and Madelin (1987).

global deforestation, legislation banning the burning of straw and a need to find alternative uses for the latter have promoted an increase in interest in effective methods of cleaning straw. One of the most promising avenues to date involves chopping and sieving processes. While these products are in current use in poultry houses, it must be emphasized that it is this author's experience that many of these products have not been efficiently or effectively cleaned and high levels of dust can be released with their use. Further work needs to be carried out to ensure the efficacy and reliability of the cleaning processes.

Careful attention to the management of bedding with frequent turning and the removal of urine and faeces is important, especially in warm weather. Under these management conditions in a well-ventilated stable, fungal growth in plant-based beddings should be prevented. Dampening of dry woodshaving beddings decreases the release of respirable dust, though woodshavings and other non-treated biological beddings must be kept dry in storage before they are used or contamination with fungi will occur before bedding down. Future research into the use of fungal inhibitors, such as weak thiabendazole solutions, will be of particular benefit in preventing the moulding of plant-based materials in stables. Non-biological and treated beddings should allay such risks.

Attention to the bedding of horses is often neglected in their convalescence after surgery or illness. Horses lying on a straw or shavings bedding, for example, have their nostrils positioned for maximum pathogen uptake. Horses with pulmonary oedema after an anaesthetic and pneumonic foals in a deep, warm straw bedding, may inhale millions of spores per minute into an already compromised respiratory system. Failure to use the alternative beddings in such situations seems inexcusable.

Rotting mounds of used beddings provide another source of potential pathogens. These mounds are often placed at the back of stables in close proximity to vents. Such mounds should be avoided near stables. Used bedding is best placed in a skip or trailer and removed from the close proximity to stables at least every third day.

CONCLUSION

The horse is long-lived compared with other species of agricultural animals and its production, i.e. athletic ability, is more closely linked to respiratory well-being than with other species. Initial stages of respiratory diseases are therefore likely to be manifested as decreased performance in early life with more severe clinical disease becoming more apparent in later life. Optimal air hygiene for horses involves attention to the macroenvironment of the stable or barn as a whole, particularly in relation to ventilation and thorough mixing of air within the building. Microenvironments surrounding the hay net or close to bedding must also be considered. A horse eating from a hay net containing mouldy hay or sniffing at a contaminated bedding may inhale a pathogenic challenge in spite of very efficient ventilation of its housing.

ACKNOWLEDGEMENTS

The author is indebted to the Home of Rest for Horses which generously sponsored a 3-year study on air hygiene and chronic pulmonary disease in the horse.

REFERENCES AND FURTHER READING

Asquith, R. L. (1983). *Aflatoxin and Aspergillus Flavus in Corn*, p.62. Alabama, Auburn University.

Bruce, J. M. (1981). *Environmental Aspects of Housing for Animal Production* (ed. J. A. Clark) p.197. London, Butterworth.

Burrell, M. H. (1985). *The Animal Health Trust Annual Report*, p. 54.

Burrell, M. H., Mackintosh, M. E., Whitwell, K. E., Mumford, J. A. & Rossdale, P. D. (1985). *Proceedings of the Society of Veterinary Epidemiology and Preventive Medicine*, p.74.

Clarke, A. F. (1987a) *Equine Veterinary Journal* **19**, 435.

Clarke, A. F. (1987b) In Hickman's *Horse Management*, p.125. Academic Press, London.

Clark, A. F. & Madelin, T. M. (1987). *Equine Veterinary Journal* **19**, 442.

Clarke, A. F., Madelin, T. M. & Allpress, R. G. (1987). *Equine Veterinary Journal* **19**(6), 524.

Cuddeford, D. (1986). Veterinary Record Supplement *In Practice* **8**, 68.

Derksen, F. J. *et al. Journal of Applied Physiology* **58**, 598.

Donaldson, (1978). *The Veterinary Bulletin* **48**, 83.

Enarson, D., Vedal, S. & Change-Yeung, M. (1985). *American Review of Respiratory Disease* **132**, 814.

Gregory, P. H., Lacey, M. E., Festenstein, G. N. & Skinner, F. A. (1963). *Journal of Microbiology* **33**, 147.

Jones, R. D., McGreevy, P. C., Robertson, A., Clarke, A. F. & Wathes, C. M. (1987). *Equine Veterinary Journal* **19**, 454.

Lacey, J., Lord, K. A., King, H. G. & Manlove, R. (1978). *Annals of Applied Biology* **88**, 65.

McCormack, J. A. O., Clark, J. J. & Knowles, L. C. (1984). *Farm Building Progress* **78**, 31.

McPherson, E. A., Lawson, G. H., Murphy, J. R., Nicholson, J. M., Breeze, R. G. & Pirie, H. M. (1978). *Equine Veterinary Journal* **10**, 47.

Percivall, W. (1853). *The Diseases of the Chest and Air Passage of the Horse*, London, Longman Brown Green & Longmans.

Sainsbury, D. W. B. (1981). *Equine Veterinary Journal* **13**, 167.

CHAPTER 5

Tracheostomy

PATRICK DIXON

INTRODUCTION

Tracheostomy refers to an artificial opening into the trachea and is usually taken to include the use of a tracheostomy tube to keep this opening patent. Tracheotomy is the surgical procedure of creating a tracheostomy, although some authors use these words interchangeably. The benefits of such were recognized early on;

> The respiratory canal is occasionally obstructed, to an annoying and dangerous degree. It has been anxiously inquired whether there might not be established an artificial opening for the passage of the air, when the natural one could no longer be used. It has now been ascertained that it is both a simple and safe operation.

> *The Horse* by William Youatt, New Edition 1846.

Temporary tracheostomy

A tracheostomy tube is inserted, usually for a matter of days, because an acute upper airflow obstruction is present or anticipated, e.g. severe upper respiratory infection causing laryngeal oedema.

Permanent tracheostomy

A tracheostomy tube is used to bypass a permanent upper airway obstruction. A permanent tracheostomy is most commonly used in performance animals to bypass performance limiting less severe respiratory obstruction, e.g. cases of laryngeal paralysis non responsive to conventional surgery. The term permanent tracheostomy is not absolute because for ease of management many owners request the removal of "permanent" tracheostomy tubes at the end of each working season, with its replacement at the beginning of the following season.

The horse has a large relatively superficial trachea which facilitates tracheotomy. It tolerates a tracheostomy tube in situ very well, with very little coughing, due to the low sensitivity of the equine trachea. After a few days postoperative inflammation, relatively little blockage of the tube with exudate and normal respiratory secretions occurs in equines, compared to other species. Nevertheless there will always be some residual discharge around a tracheostomy particularly if the animal has chronic pulmonary disease and some owners find this aesthetically objectionable.

INDICATIONS FOR TEMPORARY TRACHEOSTOMY

Acute upper respiratory obstructions

Severe upper respiratory obstruction presents as an anxious, sweating horse with possibly stridorous breathing noises at rest, flared nostrils, extended neck, increased costo-abdominal respiratory effort, cyanosis and functioning accessory muscles of respiration. Particularly if the last two signs are present, a temporary tracheostomy is imperative.

This type of obstruction can be caused by severe acute upper respiratory infections, e.g. strangles or cellulitis or, much less commonly, by viral infections. It may also occur after anaphylactoid reactions such as insect stings or due to post injection reactions (Fig. 5.1) or infections in the neck region. Trauma to the head or throat region may also cause inflammation and oedema severe enough to necessitate tracheostomy.

After major upper respiratory surgery

After major upper respiratory surgery such as bilateral arytenoidectomy or after postoperative bilateral nasal packing to control haemorrhage, prophylactic tracheostomy is indicated. Temporary tracheostomies are usually unnecessary after ventriculectomy or laryngoplasty unless postoperative inflammation occurs to such a degree as to obstruct the laryngeal cavity. Under these very rare circumstances a temporary tracheostomy tube can be inserted through the laryngotomy wound, if present, or through the usual tracheal sites. However the routine use of temporary tracheostomy tubes at this site should not be performed as these tubes always cause local irritation and secondary infection of the adjacent respiratory mucosa and delayed healing of the laryngotomy wound occurs. Indeed contrary to popular belief, routine laryngotomy wounds can safely have the laryngeal mucosa sutured, allowing rapid healing of the wound due to the absence of its continuous contamination by respiratory secretions and exudate.

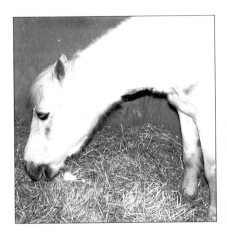

Fig. 5.1
A pony with marked head and neck oedema caused by an adverse injection reaction in the neck. Laryngeal and perilaryngeal oedema are now causing severe respiratory embarrassment. The animal is distressed, with its head extended and making loud stridorous noises. It cannot fully flare its oedematous nostrils. The neck has been clipped for a temporary tracheostomy.

Inhalation anaesthesia

A tracheostomy can be used to permit inhalation anaesthesia during major head surgery, e.g. arytenoidectomy.

Bronchoscopy

A distal tracheostomy allows examination of the more distal smaller airways with a smaller diameter, shorter endoscope (Fig. 5.2).

INDICATIONS FOR PERMANENT TRACHEOSTOMY

Permanent severe upper respiratory obstructions

Bilateral facial paralysis presents a case for permanent tracheostomy, as the horse is an obligate nasal breather. Inoperable nasal and sinus neoplasia or ethmoid haematomas may also be treated in the short term, e.g. to allow a pregnant mare to foal.

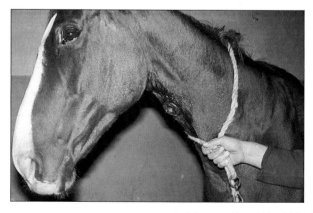

Fig. 5.2 Steeplechaser suffering from mild bilateral nasal paralysis, caused by a bitless bridle, 24 h after the insertion of a permanent tracheostomy tube. Note the limited degree of postoperative inflammation at this site.

Tracheal obstruction

Permanent tracheostomy is indicated for such as scabbard trachea, i.e. lateral flattening. This occurs usually in larger horses, is most severe cranially and is therefore amenable to a distal tracheostomy (Fig. 5.3). Dorsoventral flattening usually occurs in small ponies and commonly involves the distal and intrathoracic trachea and so are usually unsuitable for tracheostomy (Figs. 5.4 and 5.5).

Acquired tracheal obstructions include trauma with rupture of tracheal rings, inversion and transected tracheal rings after tracheostomy or post tracheostomy granulomas.

Less severe airway obstruction in performance animals

Cases of laryngeal paralysis or soft palate subluxation may not be responsive to conventional surgery. In this latter instance particularly, a tracheostomy can also be used prior to any surgery to assess if the alleged airway obstruction is a primary performance limiting factor or just a non-specific

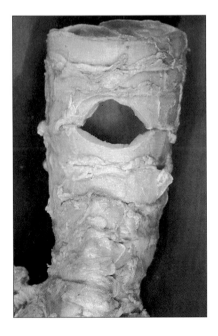

Fig. 5.3
Tracheal specimen from a thoroughbred with lateral flattening of the anterior tracheal rings. Distal to this obstruction parts of two adjacent tracheal rings have been removed which would allow a permanent tracheostomy at this site.

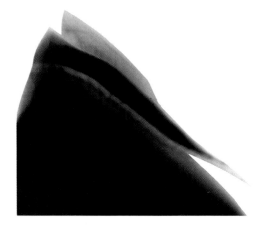

Fig. 5.4
Lateral radiograph of a Shetland pony
which showed severe respiratory
distress even at rest. Dorsoventral
collapse of the distal cervical trachea
is present.

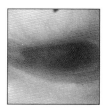

Fig. 5.5
Endoscopic view of dorsoventral tracheal collapse in a pony.

sign of exhaustion. Some countries, like USA, do not allow racehorses to run with tracheostomies and in general this treatment is less commonly performed nowadays. It is unclear if the unfiltered, unhumidified and unheated air entering the trachea at right angles from a tracheostomy has any adverse effects on pulmonary function.

SURGICAL ANATOMY AND PROCEDURE

The normal anatomical features and surgical technique required for this procedure should be understood in advance as temporary tracheostomy is frequently an emergency procedure, with little time to consult a reference. Anatomical details of the upper cervical trachea are shown in Figs 5.6 and 5.7. It can be seen that there are no vital structures overlying the anterior aspect of the cervical trachea.

The procedure is usually carried out on the standing animal under local anaesthesia. In any case many animals requiring a temporary tracheostomy would not survive general anaesthesia. Unless the airflow obstruction is in the cervical trachea, the usual tracheostomy site is the upper third of the cervical trachea, commonly at the third to the fifth tracheal rings. This site has advantages in that the trachea is most superficial here. Moreover, if tracheostomy induced granulation tissue eventually causes a tracheal obstruction, one can reoperate on the animal distally. The tube is also less likely to get caught or rubbed on doors or gates at this level as compared to the lower neck.

A midline area 15 cm long and 7 cm wide overlying the chosen tracheal site is shaved and the skin prepared for surgery; 20 ml of local anaesthetic is infiltrated midline subcutaneously and into the underlying muscles. The animal's head is then extended to make the trachea more prominent, provided that this manipulation does not worsen the dyspnoea in animals with gross laryngeal obstructions. A 7 cm midline skin incision will expose the underlying cutaneous colli muscle, which is also transected midline. If present, small skin bleeding points should be controlled with haemostats. It is

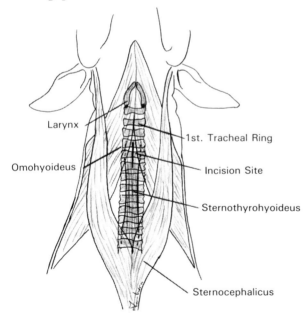

Larynx

1st. Tracheal Ring

Omohyoideus

Incision Site

Sternothyrohyoideus

Sternocephalicus

Fig. 5.6
Diagram of ventral aspect of equine neck with tracheostomy site indicated.

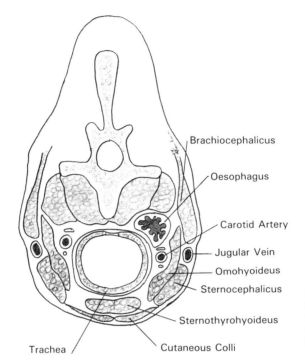

Brachiocephalicus

Oesophagus

Carotid Artery

Jugular Vein

Omohyoideus

Sternocephalicus

Sternothyrohyoideus

Cutaneous Colli

Trachea

Fig. 5.7
Diagram of cross
section of equine
neck at the 4th
tracheal ring.

helpful if an assistant laterally retracts the cutaneous colli muscle and skin, with tissue forceps, to reveal the under-lying sternothyrohyoideus muscles. The ill-defined junction between the paired bodies of these muscles can be identified as a fine fibrous line which can usually be avascularly divided with scissors. Separation of these muscles will now reveal the trachea to which they are loosely attached by a minimum of connective tissue and laterally the paired omohyoideus muscles. These latter muscles should be bluntly dissected off the trachea to expose its anterior surface.

In emergency cases there may not be time to follow the above procedures and one may have to, without skin preparation or anaesthesia, make a deep midline incision down to the tracheal surface.

TEMPORARY TRACHEOSTOMY

A transverse stab incision is made into the most distal annular ligament exposed. With scissors, this incision is extended on both sides to create an opening large enough for the temporary tracheostomy tube. This incision should not be continued more than halfway through the circumference of the annular ligament in case the carotid artery or associated nerves are transected. The temporary tracheostomy tube (Fig. 5.8) is then manipulated through this opening and down the trachea. If a temporary tracheostomy tube is unavailable, one can readily be fashioned from a plastic container handle or piece of stomach tube, with holes drilled or burned into them to allow them to be taped or sutured to the neck (Fig. 5.9). It is helpful to insert two heavy monofilament nylon suture loops, 6 in long encircling the tracheal rings above and below the incision. With moderate traction on these loops, the tracheal incision can be dilated to facilitate tube reinsertion after cleaning and minimizing the risk of its accidental insertion down a fascial plane anterior to the trachea by inexperienced owners.

PERMANENT TRACHEOSTOMY

Because the narrow annular rings in the horse are not wide enough to accommodate the much larger permanent tracheostomy tubes (Fig 5.10) parts of two adjacent tracheal

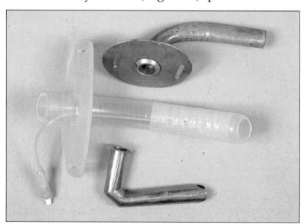

Fig. 5.8
Two metal equine temporary tracheostomy tubes and a modern plastic cuffed temporary tracheostomy tube. Where this latter type is used with the cuff inflated it is even more critical that its lumen be cleaned frequently.

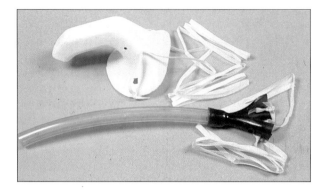

Fig. 5.9
Two examples of makeshift temporary tracheostomy tubes. One is made from a stomach tube and one from the handle of a plastic container.

rings (as shown in Figure 5.6) and very occasionally the complete anterior aspect of one ring will have to be removed. Various designs of tracheotomes, i.e. instruments for removing portions of tracheal rings, were once commonly used but are not readily available nowadays. This procedure can be equally well performed by grasping the tracheal ring firmly through the annular ligament stab incision with a large artery forceps and making a semi-lunar incision with a solid scalpel or with heavy curved scissors. A firm grip should be maintained on the tracheal ring both to allow proper control of the incision and to prevent inhalation of the excised piece of cartilage.

One should avoid cutting fully through a tracheal ring because after the tracheostomy tube removal, the transected ends may invert into and partially occlude the tracheal lumen,

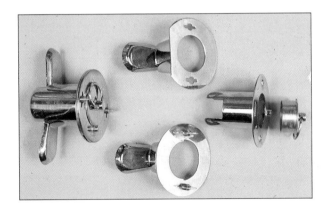

Fig. 5.10
A dismantled and an assembled permanent tracheostomy tube.

particularly if two or more rings are transected (Fig. 5.11). This is mainly a problem in foals where a temporary tracheostomy has been attempted using an adult sized temporary tracheostomy tube which has been found to be too large to fit through an annular space, with subsequent transection of a number of tracheal rings to enable its insertion.

AFTER CARE

Temporary tracheostomy

Depending on its immune status, the animal should be given tetanus antitoxin. A broad spectrum antibiotic should be given for 3–4 days as it will decrease the inevitable postoperative local infection that develops and so lessen the exudate that causes the major problem in the first few days postoperatively due to tube blockage. It is imperative that the tube's lumen be kept patent, otherwise the blocked tracheostomy tube will act as an additional obstruction and so worsen the animal's airflow (Fig. 5.12). Temporary tracheostomy tubes need to be cleaned three to four times the first day and twice daily after that.

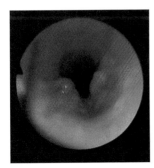

Fig. 5.11
Endoscopic view of post tracheostomy stenosis which has been caused by complete transection of two tracheal rings during a previous tracheostomy.

With temporary tracheostomies it is very helpful if a spare temporary tube is available so that they can be changed over for cleaning. After removal of the tube, soaking in detergent and the use of a wire bottle brush, followed by thorough rinsing in water is effective. The skin beneath the tracheostomy should be coated in Vaseline to prevent skin excoriation and facilitate skin cleaning. Animals are best kept indoors in a box where they cannot rub and possibly dislodge the tube. After the primary respiratory obstruction is resolved and the temporary tracheostomy tube and the two nylon loops are removed, the tracheostomy wound, which is inevitably contaminated, should not be sutured but should be allowed to heal by secondary intention (Fig. 5.13).

Permanent tracheostomy

Particularly if it has to be performed lower down the neck, where there is greater muscle cover by the sternocephalicus and also the larger, and at this site separate bodies of the sternothyroideus and sternohyoideus muscles, postoperative inflammation can cause complications (Fig. 5.14). The inevitable postoperative swelling of the tissues overlying the trachea can cause such pressure on the tube that it cannot be removed for cleaning without great force. It can also cause great pressure by the internal flange of the tube on the tracheal mucosa, which can lead to pressure necrosis. This is a reason for the development of tracheal granulation tissue (Fig. 5.15), which can in time cause a new airway obstruction. This inflammation can also cause great pressure on the skin by the external flange of the tube and can even cause the flange to sink below the

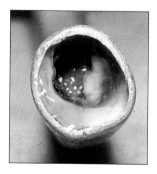

Fig. 5.12
View of the distal end of a tracheostomy tube showing almost total blockage of the lumen with respiratory exudates. In a cuffed tube this degree of blockage would prove fatal.

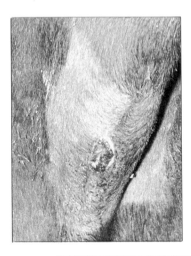

Fig. 5.13
Distal temporary tracheostomy site used for bronchoscopy 7
days previously. The wound is healing normally by
secondary intention.

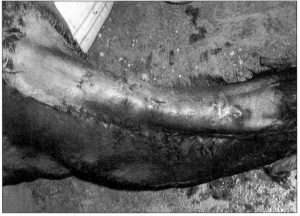

Fig. 5.14 Ventral aspect of neck of 5-year-old thoroughbred racehorse showing scarring where "permanent"
tracheostomies have been performed sequentially down the neck because of recurrent post tracheostomy stenosis.

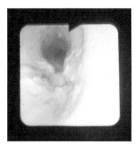

Fig. 5.15
Endoscopic view of post tracheostomy stenosis caused by granulation
tissue.

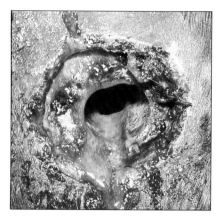

Fig. 5.16
Racehorse which had a low permanent
tracheostomy 2 weeks previously. The postoperative
inflammation has been so great that the external
flange of the permanent tracheostomy tube is now
lying subcutaneously.

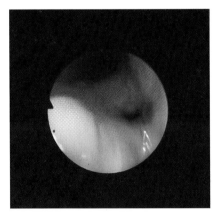

Fig. 5.17
Endoscopic view of proximal trachea of a hunter
with a tracheal fistula, 2 months after removal of the
"permanent" tracheostomy tube. The dark
mucocutaneous junction is visible on the right.

skin surface (Fig. 5.16) and eventually get totally embedded
in scar tissue. If possible, a longer necked permanent tracheostomy tube of the same diameter, which can accommodate the
tissue swelling without causing undue pressure on the tracheal
mucosa or skin surface, should be used for the first 2 weeks
postoperatively. In some animals one may have to resort to
removal of sections of these overlying muscles, before fitting
the tube.

The removal for cleaning of permanent tracheostomy tubes
by owners who have little regard for the gentle and hygienic
handling of tissues can be another factor in the exacerbation
of postoperative inflammation and the development of intratra-
cheal granulomas. After permanent tracheostomy the surgeon

should, if possible, remove and fully clean the tube daily for the first few days and after that instruct the owner how to clean it in situ daily with a blunt ended blade, such as a round ended table knife. Animals that have been shown to develop tracheal granuloma formation, should not have their tubes removed for cleaning at any stage, with all cleaning in situ. In all cases where a permanent tube is removed for cleaning, it should be replaced as quickly as possible, as local inflammation can make replacement impossible even within a few hours.

If a permanent tube is removed at the end of a season's work or on retiral to stud, the wound will normally heal over fully within weeks. If full healing does not occur, this usually indicates the development of continuity between the tracheal mucosa and skin, i.e. tracheal fistula (Fig. 5.17). This can be generally treated by freshening up the edges of the fistula.

ACKNOWLEDGEMENTS

To colleagues in practice who referred these cases, Mr R. Munro for photography, M. Camburn for the line drawings and Mrs C. Brown and Mrs M. Nicol for typing the manuscript.

REFERENCES AND FURTHER READING

Haynes, P. F. (1984). Surgery of the equine respiratory tract. In *The Practice of Large Animal Surgery*, Vol. 1 (ed. P. B. Jennings). Philadelphia, W. B. Saunders.

O'Connor, J. J. (1950). *Dollar's Veterinary Surgery*, 4th Edn. pp.308–314. London, Baillière, Tindall & Cox.

Share-Jones, J. T. (1908). *The Surgical Anatomy of the Horse*, Part 1, pp.73–77. London, Baillière, Tindall & Cox.

Wooldridge, G. H. (1928). *Encyclopaedia of Veterinary Medicine, Surgery and Obstetrics*, Vol. II, pp.949–954. London, Henry Frowde, Hodder & Stoughton.

CHAPTER 6

Grass Sickness

JOHN S. GILMOUR

INTRODUCTION

Grass sickness continues to be a serious threat to equine health and welfare in Britain, feared more in some regions than in others but liable to strike wherever equidae are kept. Thus new information of practical value to veterinary surgeons faced with the disease is a much-sought commodity. Significant advances in grass sickness research have been made since 1955 but many of these, while having great fundamental value, offer little or no assistance to the practitioner faced with the harsh reality. This article deals mainly with diagnosis and epidemiology, presenting selected information of practical value and, as the question "what is being done about it?" is a common one, also summarizes current grass sickness research objectives.

DIAGNOSIS

GENERAL OBSERVATIONS

In the absence of a reliable diagnostic test in the living animal, the diagnosis of grass sickness continues to present the equine clinician with considerable problems. At present, the ultimate diagnosis depends upon the demonstration of characteristic neuronal changes in the autonomic ganglia. Exploratory laparotomy and even gross post mortem findings are not necessarily diagnostic. Many of the clinical signs associated with the disease, particularly in its more acute form, are shared with other predominantly, but not exclusively, alimentary conditions. These conditions, together with their differentiating features, are shown in Table 6.1.

A small survey (unpublished) carried out by Dr D. Doxey and colleagues in the Department of Veterinary Clinical Studies, Royal (Dick) School of Veterinary Studies, in which 26 referred cases were followed to a conclusion, serves to illustrate some of the practical problems. An initial diagnosis of grass sickness was made in 14 cases, intestinal obstruction in eight, and uncertainty remained in four. At necropsy grass sickness was confirmed in 10 of the 14, in four of the obstructions and in one of the "uncertains". Close analysis revealed that 12% of typically acute cases and 40% of typically chronic cases (on initial assessment) were not grass sickness. Atypical initial signs had been seen in 30% of both acute and chronic cases.

There is no effective treatment for grass sickness. Acute cases can be maintained by decompression of the stomach via a nasogastric tube three times a day together with frequent intravenous fluid therapy, but death will occur once this is discontinued. At present we have no alternative but to destroy humanely any horse with grass sickness as soon as the diagnosis is certain – or as certain as it can be in the live animal.

Table 6.1 Conditions most likely to be confused with grass sickness and the features which might differentiate them.

Conditions	Features used in differentiating from grass sickness
Obstruction of small intestine	Severe unrelenting pain with violent behaviour. Bowel sounds progressively reduced. Rectal examination: palpation of distended loops of intestine and perhaps an obstructing mass. Thickened and rubbery if infarcted. Abdominocentesis: in necrotic conditions, serosanguinous becoming "muddy".
Obstruction of large intestine	
(a) Impaction	Slow in onset. Small intestinal sounds not abolished. Rectal examination: the colon is evenly distended rather than corrugated as in grass sickness.
(b) Volvulus, herniation or infarction	Severe, unrelenting pain, fever and brick red mucous membranes. Rectal examination: if infarcted, thickened and rubbery. Abdominocentesis: turbid, sanguinous, neutrophils.
Gastric dilatation	
(a) Primary	History of access to excess concentrates or fermentable foodstuff. Rapid circulatory collapse. If caused by air, relieved by stomach tube.
(b) Secondary	See obstruction of small intestine.
Verminous arteritis leading to thromboembolic colic	Rectal examination: pain on palpating coeliaco-mesenteric artery. Abdominocentesis: protein elevated followed by rise in white cell numbers. Red cells and bacteria if infarction occurs
Peritonitis	Rigid abdomen. Abdominocentesis: turbid, rise in protein and white cell numbers. May be bacteria.
Abdominal haemorrhage	Abdominocentesis: pure blood.
"Anterior enteritis"	Pyrexia. Sometimes occult blood in the gastric fluid.
Chronic nephritis/pyelonephritis	Urine: blood-tinged, elevated protein, neutrophils, bacteria. Rectal examination: dilated painful ureters and roughened renal surfaces.
Helminthiasis	Regular diarrhoea Faecal egg counts response to anthelmintic treatment.

CLINICAL SIGNS

Grass sickness occurs in peracute, acute, subacute and chronic forms, all of which are generally regarded as representing differing degrees in the manifestation of one essential pathological condition. It has been customary to make this classification on the basis of the severity of signs and how soon the horse dies. The condition is basically a neurogenic obstruction of the alimentary tract, which may be partial or complete, and involves various parts of the tract to differing degrees. Consequently it is not surprising that there are considerable individual variations in the clinical picture.

PERACUTE/ACUTE GRASS SICKNESS

Peracute/acute grass sickness (defined as illness leading to death in less than 2 days) may be suspected on detection of several of the following signs.

(1)   The animal is very depressed.
(2)   The pulse rate is accelerated to 70–80/min, sometimes rising above 100/min.
(3)   There is complete bowel stasis and atony from pharynx to rectum.
(4)   Borborygmi are absent.
(5)   Abdominal distension may be evident and tympani can be detected on auscultation and percussion.
(6)   The grossly distended stomach may contain in excess of 20 l of fluid.
(7)   Greenish, mucinous, watery stomach contents are regurgitated into the pharynx and mouth, and may be forcibly ejected from the nose.
(8)   Gastric rupture may occur.
(9)   Variable amounts of thick glairy saliva are drooled from the mouth.
(10)   Swallowing is difficult and painful, and can stimulate reverse peristalsis in the oesophagus.
(11)   Abdominal pain, which can be severe, is sometimes evident.
(12)   Patchy sweating is seen behind the shoulders and on the flanks typically.

(13)   Fine muscular tremors occur, especially over the triceps, hip and stifle areas.

Evidence of colic appears to be a particularly poor guide to a diagnosis and care must be exercised if examination follows analgesic treatment, particularly when flunixin meglumine has been administered. This drug is particularly effective not only in abolishing acute pain but in masking the endotoxin-induced cardiovascular derangements resulting from ischaemic obstruction of bowel, so producing a state of depression similar to that of the grass sickness patient.

On rectal examination, normal faeces are absent and the rectal mucosa is dry and tacky. Small balls of hard faeces are closely adherent to the mucosa. The colon contains firm material often clearly in excess, and distended, fluid-filled loops of small intestine may be palpated extending back towards the pelvic inlet.

SUBACUTE/CHRONIC GRASS SICKNESS

Subacute cases of grass sickness die usually within a week or two of the onset of signs while chronic cases can linger for months. The clinical signs are of lowish grade and degrees of large intestinal stasis are quite apparent. Transition from health to illness can be insidious, particularly in chronic cases. Weight loss, patch sweating and intermittent colic are often the first signs noticed. The animal is dull and may wander restlessly. Muscular tremors may be present intermittently. Attempts to eat and drink are often followed by regurgitation down the nose. If a horse succeeds in swallowing, abdominal pain may follow within minutes. Defaecation is infrequent and the faeces are scanty and hard. In affected geldings the penis is often pendulous. A degree of jaundice is not uncommon, but the most striking feature is the dramatic loss of physical condition, accompanied by muscle atrophy and dehydration. The abdomen is tucked up to an exaggerated degree, giving the appearance of an emaciated greyhound. Death eventually ocurs from cachexia, debility and exhaustion if the horse is not destroyed on humane grounds.

AIDS TO DIAGNOSIS

Laboratory aids

There is no laboratory test providing confirmation of grass sickness in vivo. Serum protein alterations occur, but do not specifically identify the disease. Plasma catecholamines which have been shown to be present in markedly higher concentration in grass sickness cases than in normal horses or in those with obstructive colic (Hodson et al., 1984) may prove of value in diagnosis. However, their measurement is complex, expensive and currently not widely available.

Abdominocentesis

Peritoneal fluid, which is often reduced in volume in grass sickness, is macroscopically normal in appearance but usually contains increased protein – normal range 0·1–3·4 g/dl (Bach and Ricketts, 1974). Furthermore, the absence of red blood cells helps to eliminate a strangulating obstruction of the intestine.

Barium swallow

Using image intensification radiography, this is of value in assessing oesophageal motility. In 18 cases of grass sickness, one or other of two types of swallowing defect was observed, although this could also indicate a non-specific neurological impairment (Greet and Whitwell, 1986).

Laparotomy

When any doubt remains about the diagnosis in a horse suspected of having grass sickness, an exploratory laparotomy to eliminate a physical obstruction which might be corrected surgically is justified. However, it is not uncommon to find secondary ileal impaction resulting from impaired gut motility, or malpositions of the large colon in horses with grass sickness. In these cases, clearing the impaction or replacing the colon in its correct position will not bring about recovery.

POST-MORTEM FINDINGS

Confirmation of diagnosis in grass sickness rests upon post-mortem examinations. Grossly, acute and subacute cases may show characteristically hard, dry, dark-coated colonic and caecal contents (Fig. 6.1). Variably large volumes of foul-smelling gastric liquid are present, though occasionally the organ has ruptured before necropsy. Chronic cases are usually remarkable only for the degree of weight loss.

In order to confirm a diagnosis of grass sickness, histological examination of peripheral autonomic ganglia, brain and spinal cord is required (Fig. 6.2). When facilities for full necropsy are not available and experience in locating ganglia is lacking, submission of 20–30 cm of a thoracic sympathetic chain of ganglia is sufficient. This structure is readily visible through the pleura in reasonably fresh carcases, as two flat bands of nerve fibres, 4–10 mm wide, running parallel to the spine, one on either side of the ventral surface of the thoracic vertebral bodies and 5–10 cm distant from the midline depending on the size of the animal. Careful dissection will include a 2–3 mm nodule of ganglion tissue at each intercostal interval and the

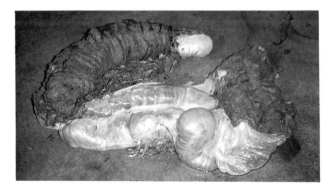

Fig. 6.1 Hard, dry, dark-covered contents in caecum and colon at necropsy of an acute case of grass sickness.

section removed should be fixed in 10% formol saline for laboratory examination.

EPIDEMIOLOGY AND PREVENTION

Grass sickness has been confirmed in all species of equidae in Britain, not only horses and ponies, but donkeys, zebras and Przewalski's horse.

Although the disease may be rare in some regions, it has been confirmed in every area of England and Wales, and in Scotland, except the extreme north west. Recent reports from Ireland are not available, but grass sickness was convincingly described in that country in the 1940s, thus may still occur.

Results from the only survey which produced real prevalence statistics (Gilmour and Jolly, 1974) are given in Table 6.2.

Dr Doxey's survey confirmed the observations in Table 6.2 and adds the statistic that at least 75% of victims in a series of 100 had been subjected to some major change in management shortly before the illness.

On statistical grounds, animals in category A in the table comprise a "high risk" population and may be selected for stabling in an effort to reduce that risk. In animals stabled overnight, or for part of the day, grass sickness occurred with an infrequency similar to that in solely stabled animals, therefore a basis exists for rational attempts to avoid the disease.

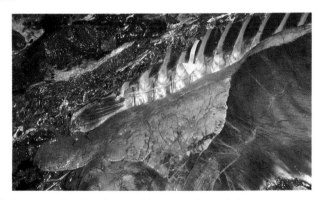

Fig. 6.2 Equine necropsy: thoracic cavity exposed by removal of one wall. Arrow shows a thoracic sympathetic chain of ganglia.

Table 6.2 Prevalence of grass sickness.

A. Grass sickness significantly associated with:
    2- to 7-year-old animals
    Equidae kept solely out of doors
    March to June
    Recently-arrived stock
    Premises where grass sickness has
    previously occurred
B. Grass sickness not significantly associated
    with:
    Contact with an affected animal
    Particular types of grazing
    Supplementary feeding
    Breed
    Sex

Animals which have recently arrived on a premises are particularly at risk, and mares arriving at stud or returning therefrom must be included in this category. Without knowing the reason for this increased risk, it can only be suggested that part-stabling of such animals be practised for several weeks as part of providing a stress-free transition to the new environment.

SUMMARY OF RESEARCH

Recent research, other than the barium swallow studies described above, has been directed towards fundamental rather than practical aspects of the disease. Further definition of the pathogenesis is probably required in order to progress towards identification of the cause of the disease, to provide diagnostic tests and to establish specific means of prevention or cure.

In the past 13 years the following new information has been documented:

(1) A neurotoxic factor is present in serum from acute cases (Gilmour and Mould, 1977).
(2) A small molecule unique to neurotoxic serum can be demonstrated (Johnson, 1985).

(3)   Certain neuropeptides are deficient in the intestinal nerve plexuses (Bishop *et al.*, 1984).
(4)   Serum protein is altered (Johnson *et al.*, 1983).
(5)   Plasma catecholamines are increased (Hodson *et al.*, 1986).

Current collaborative research at Moredun Research Institute and the Department of Veterinary Clinical Studies in the Royal (Dick) School of Veterinary Studies seeks to identify the neurotoxic factor in serum, to define alterations to neurotransmitters in the autonomic ganglia and to serum proteins, and to carry out a survey of ingested fungi, accompanied by ongoing epidemiological studies including referred clinical cases. Most recently, one of the team, Dr Milne, has commenced research into the possibility of improving gut motility in chronic cases. A second research study is being conducted in the surgery department of Glasgow University Veterinary School where researchers are examining in depth the functional deficit in the neurological lesion in grass sickness and aim to develop a tissue culture system for study of the lesion and its reproduction.

REFERENCES AND FURTHER READING

Bach, L. G. & Ricketts, S. W. (1974). *Equine Veterinary Journal* **6**, 116.
Bishop, A. E., Hodson, N. P., Major, J. M., Probert, L., Yeats, J., Edwards, G. B., Wright, J. A., Bloom, S. A. & Polar, J. M. (1984). *Experientia* **40**, 801–806.
Gilmour, J. S. & Jolly, G. M. (1974). *Veterinary Record* **95**, 77–81.
Gilmour, J. S. & Mould, D. L. (1977). *Research in Veterinary Science* **22**, 1–4.
Greet, T. R. C. & Whitwell, K. E. (1986). *Equine Veterinary Journal* **18**, 294–297.
Hodson, N. P., Cawson, R. & Edwards, G. B. (1984). *Veterinary Record* **115**, 18.
Hodson, N. P. Wright J. A. & Hunt, J. (1986). *Veterinary Record* **118**, 148–150.
Johnson, P. (1985) *Research in Veterinary Science* **38**, 329–333.
Johnson, P., Dawson, A. McL & Mould, D. L. (1983). *Research in Veterinary Science* **35**, 165–170.

CHAPTER 7

Nasogastric Intubation

KEN URQUHART

INTRODUCTION

Nasogastric intubation or stomach tubing of horses has both diagnostic and therapeutic indications. It is not a difficult procedure provided one has a reasonably tractable patient, the correct equipment and adequate restraint.

EQUIPMENT

Nasogastric tubes come in a variety of specifications according to the type of equine (foal, pony, horse) for which they are intended and selection should consider the following.

External diameter

The diameter of the tube should be slightly less than the minimum width of the horse's ventral nasal meatus. It is wise to err on the conservative side as some horses have an unusually narrow ventral meatus. It is always possible to use a small tube in a big horse, but not vice versa.

Pliability

Soft tubes with poor rigidity should be avoided as these may become excessively pliable and difficult to pass in warm weather. More rigid tubes are easier to pass and although these may become excessively stiff in cold weather, they can be softened by immersion in warm water.

Length

The tube to be used should be sufficiently long to allow its distal end to be placed in the stomach while enough is left in reserve at the proximal end to allow the attachment of a stomach pump at ground level.

Colour

Transparent tubes allow one to see what is going down or, more importantly, coming up the tube.

RESTRAINT

Adequate restraint and assistance are essential if nasogastric intubation is to take place safely and competently. Restrain the horse with a head collar and position its quarters in the corner of a loose box to limit backward and lateral movement. Fractious horses may need additional measures and a nose twitch or sedative may be used. The latter tends to inhibit the swallowing reflex and can be counterproductive in some cases.

While intubation is in progress the veterinary surgeon and all personnel should stand to the side of the horse to avoid injury from a rearing animal. My preference is to stand on the horse's left side with the groom behind. Alternatively, the groom can stand on the opposite side where he can be placed further forward and contribute more to restraining the horse's head. Some valorous practitioners perform intubation while standing directly in front of the horse and accept the increased risk of injury. I would condemn this approach even when the horse is restrained in purpose built stocks.

INTUBATION TECHNIQUE

With the veterinary surgeon standing on the horse's left side, the palm of the right hand is placed across the nasal bones just above the external nares and the head is pulled downward into ventral flexion and slightly towards the veterinary surgeon (Fig. 7.1). The right thumb is now removed from the dorsum of the nasal bones and is used to raise and evert the laminae of the alar cartilage of the left nostril. The left nostril is now fully open (Fig. 7.2).

The stomach pump should be coiled and held in the correct position (Fig. 7.3) in the left hand.

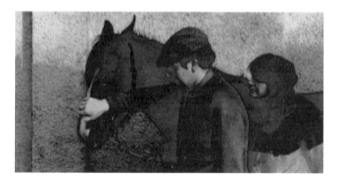

Fig. 7.1 Preliminary position with the vet standing to the horse's left side, the palm of his right hand across the nasal bones of the horse.

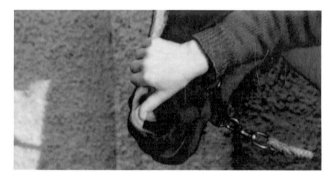

Fig. 7.2 Exposure of the left nostril with the thumb.

The first 15–25 cm of tube are now introduced gently but firmly into the ventromedial part of the left nostril where in almost every case it will enter the ventral nasal meatus (Fig. 7.4). Immediately the tube is in position, the right thumb is removed from the alar cartilage and is used to hold the tube against the nasal septum. As horses often resent this phase of intubation more than any other, it is essential that the right hand is retained in position to restrict head movement while the right thumb prevents the tube slipping out.

After the stomach tube has been introduced into the ventral meatus it is advanced 10 cm–15 cm at a time until it impinges on the pharyngeal wall and can be advanced no further. The

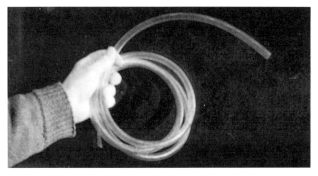

Fig. 7.3 The stomach tube is held (coiled) in the left hand with the distal 15–25 cm protruding between thumb and index finger. This portion of the tube should be well lubricated and the tip curved slightly downward.

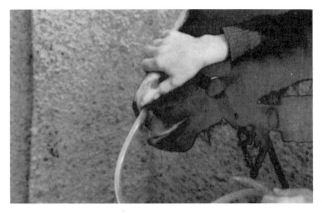

Fig. 7.4 Introduction of the stomach pump into the ventral nasal meatus.

length of tube needed to accomplish this can be gauged by prior estimation of the distance from the external nares to the pharynx (Fig. 7.5).

Where the above technique is not possible the following alternative is suggested. Standing on the horse's left side the right index finger is used to locate the ventral nasal meatus of either nostril. The stomach tube is introduced with the left hand and the tip directed below the right index finger to enter the ventral nasal meatus. The right index finger is kept firmly on top of the tube to prevent it slipping out. Although this technique seems simpler, it is more difficult to keep the head and neck flexed, and digital exploration of the nostril upsets some horses. Routine use of a nose twitch may be advisable with this method.

At this point the stomach tube cannot be advanced beyond the pharynx until the horse swallows. When swallowing occurs one must attempt to advance the tube by 15 cm–25 cm. Horses which are reluctant to swallow may be stimulated to do so by gently moving the tube in and out by a few centimetres or by syringing some water into the oral cavity.

When the tube has been passed beyond the pharynx one must ascertain whether it has entered the oesophagus or trachea before continuing. The following criteria are most reliable.

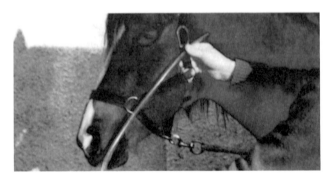

Fig. 7.5 Prior estimation of the length of tube needed in order to reach the pharynx from the external nares.

Resistance

The oesophageal wall forms a flaccid tube which creates appreciable resistance to the passage of a stomach tube. Little or no resistance is encountered in the lumen of the rigid trachea.

Aspiration of air

When suction (by mouth) is applied to the proximal end of the tube, no air can be aspirated when it is correctly placed, as the flaccid oesophageal wall occludes the side and end holes. Air can be aspirated easily and continuously if the tube lies in the trachea (Fig. 7.6).

Visualization

In most horses the tube's movement within the oesophagus is discernible as it traverses the left side of the trachea in the mid-neck region; if in doubt, the tube should be moved in and out several times to elicit further movement. Visualization may be difficult or impossible in animals which have a fat or muscular neck, heavy winter coat or a right sided oesophagus.

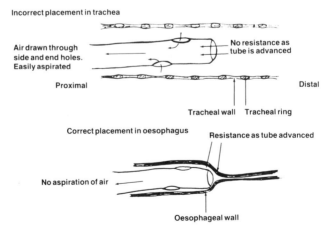

Fig. 7.6 Aspiration of air. When suction is applied to the proximal end of a correctly placed tube no air can be aspirated; air can be aspirated easily if the tube lies in the trachea.

Visual confirmation by an owner or groom who claims to have seen the tube go down should not be relied upon and should always be confirmed by the veterinary surgeon.

Release of stomach gas

When the tube is advanced into the stomach one may hear or smell a transient release of stomach gas before digesta blocks the end of the tube. To confirm this, one should blow down the tube when more gas will be released.

Other less reliable critera include:

Palpation

In thin or emaciated horses it may be possible to palpate the tube within the oesophagus. Alternatively, by vigorously shaking the larynx and trachea from side to side one may feel or hear the tube bounce off the cartilaginous wall of these organs.

Coughing

It is tempting to assume that the presence of a stomach tube within the trachea will always elicit coughing, but this is not the case, especially if the horse is twitched, sedated or depressed. Little weight should be given to the absence of coughing when assessing tube placement.

UNTOWARD SEQUELAE

Nasal haemorrhage is the most common untoward sequela to nasogastric intubation and owners should always be warned of this possibility beforehand. Haemorrhage may be profuse and it is not unusual for a horse to lose 1–2 l in the 10–15 min before spontaneous resolution occurs. To avoid this problem one should concentrate on good technique and adequate restraint and avoid the use of tubes previously used for the per-oral intubation of other species, as these frequently become abraded at their distal end and are likely to lacerate the horse's delicate and highly vascular nasal mucosa.

Cases involving the accidental deposition of therapeutic agents into the lower respiratory tract have unfortunately been recorded. This should not occur provided that one uses the above criteria to ensure that the tube is correctly placed initially and that its position is rechecked should the animal become fractious or unsettled.

CHAPTER 8

Rectal Examination of the Equine Gastrointestinal Tract

JUDITH M. HUNT

INTRODUCTION

Palpation of pelvic and abdominal structures by rectal examination in horses plays a major role in the clinical assessment of gastointestinal and urogenital disorders. This chapter concentrates on the former, providing guidance for a systematic exploration, which aids detection of abnormalities, and outlining rectal findings in some specific conditions.

TECHNIQUE

Adequate restraint is necessary to ensure the safety of both personnel and the animal: this may involve the use of a bridle or a twitch, or chemical restraint using xylazine may be preferable. If the veterinary surgeon uses the right hand for rectal examination, the horse should be positioned with the right flank against a wall and the head restrained on the left hand side. The following points should be remembered:

(1) Lubrication of the gloved hand and arm is essential.
(2) Care should be taken to ensure that no tail hairs are carried into the anus.

(3)   Considerable pressure may be required to push the hand past the anal sphincter but once this has been achieved, no further forceful action should be allowed. If the horse strains or a wave of strong contractions passes down the gut, the hand must be removed immediately.
(4)   All the faeces within reach must be removed prior to any attempt to palpate structures.
(5)   The abdominal and pelvic contents should be palpated by moving the hand along the surfaces rather than by grasping any structures through the gut wall.
(6)   At the end of any examination, the hand should be checked for blood stained faeces or frank blood.

ROUTINE EXPLORATION

In certain conditions, abnormalities of the gastrointestinal tract are apparent immediately. However, in less easily recognizable cases, the adoption of a systematic approach decreases the possibility of lesions being missed or of their significance being misunderstood. Findings in normal animals are illustrated in Figure 8.1, as are some commonly occurring abnormal findings.

Pelvis

With the exception of small colon, there should be no other gut palpable. The bladder may be distended, especially if the horse has not been given opportunities for urination. Occasionally the bladder must be emptied before palpation of more cranial structures can be performed. A gravid uterus may also hinder rectal examination.

Aorta

The aorta and the bifurcation to the external iliac vessels together with the arterial pulse can be palpated in the dorsal midline. This is a useful landmark and in some animals (depending on size and lack of straining) the course of the aorta can be followed cranially to the mesenteric root.

Mesenteric root

This presents as a structure running in a dorsoventral direction and it may be possible to detect pulsation within the tissues. There is poor correlation between apparent pain and swelling in this structure assessed by rectal examination and pathological changes caused by verminous infestation found at subsequent post mortem examination.

Left kidney

The caudal pole of the left kidney is palpable and can be located by moving the hand from the aorta around the left dorsal abdominal wall. The kidney is retroperitoneal and therefore presents as a firm swelling which cannot be separated from the body wall. (The right kidney is not palpable.) Moving laterally from the kidney it is usually possible in all except very large horses to feel the nephrosplenic ligament.

Nephrosplenic ligament

This runs transversely across the abdomen from the medial aspect of the spleen to the kidney. In the normal horse, there is no intestine palpable dorsal to this ligament.

Spleen

This can be located via the nephrosplenic ligament or by bringing the hand back to the pelvic brim and then moving cranially along the left body wall. The hand should come into contact with the caudal margin of the spleen although the position can vary greatly. At times this margin will be just cranial to the pelvis but alternatively may be palpable only at arm's reach. However, it should lie against the body wall with no intestine on its lateral surface. From the spleen, the hand

should be moved ventrally to examine the left and right
inguinal regions.

Left and right inguinal regions

These are particularly important in stallions if inguinal herniation is suspected. All intestines in this area should be
freely moveable.

Left large colon

The pelvic flexure of the colon is the junction of the left dorsal
and ventral portions and should lie immediately cranial to the
pelvic brim, in the midline or slightly to the left hand side.
This flexure has one taenial band running along the attachment
of the mesocolon. This band can be followed along the left
ventral colon, around the flexure and on to the left dorsal
colon. The band should not be under tension and the contents
of the colon should be soft and the wall relaxed.

Caecum

This can be palpated on the right side of the abdomen. The
ventral and medial taenial bands can be located as they pass
around the caudal aspect of the caecal base and body and
then run cranially towards the apex. Often it is possible to
appreciate caecal motility and gas within the viscus although
this should not be producing actual distension.

Small colon

This can be palpated in areas unoccupied by the large colon;
as it has a long mesenteric attachment its position is variable.
The major distinguishing feature, unless gut transit has been
affected, is the presence of faecal balls. The diameter of the
gut and the two taenial bands also differentiate the small from
the large colon.

Peritoneum

Both visceral and parietal peritoneum should be smooth and non-painful.

It is not possible to palpate small intestinal loops in a normal horse; the jejunum has a long mesenteric attachment and moves away from the hand. It is important to remember that it is possible to explore only 40% approximately of the abdomen by rectal palpation; thus, cranially located lesions may exist which cannot be discerned.

SPECIFIC RECTAL FINDINGS (FIG. 8.1)

IMPACTION OF THE PELVIC FLEXURE

When impacted, the pelvic flexure increases in size and, in all but mild cases, comes to lie within the pelvis. In severe cases it is palpable within 5 cm of the anal sphincter. Typically, as the hand and arm are moved cranially, the pelvic floor cannot be felt and there is an obvious mass displacing the rectum in a dorsal direction. Assessment of the nature of this distended viscus is essential. An impaction presents as a doughy mass and can be indented by manual pressure with the indentation remaining for 5–10 s. The gut wall around the impaction is smooth, taenial bands can be palpated on the more cranial portions of the left colon and the impaction often extends beyond arm's reach. Occasionally there may be some gaseous caecal distension. However, if the distended viscus within the pelvis is not compressible and the gut wall is taut and resists indentation, then gaseous distension is probable. This indicates a colonic torsion, colonic displacement or blockage of the small colon. If no taenial bands can be palpated along the cranial portion, small intestinal impaction may be present although this is a relatively rare intrapelvic rectal finding.

Secondary impaction of the pelvic flexure occurs in a number of conditions. Non-strangulating torsions or displacements result in some impairment of gut transit but additional gaseous distension and, or, oedema of the gut wall or mesocolon (gelatinous or rubbery feel) are often present. Colonic stasis (e.g. in chronic grass disease) or hypovolaemia can result in absorption of fluid from the colon and the remaining firm ingesta may be mistaken for an impaction. The major differentiating factor is that the gut wall appears corrugated as it follows the outline of the contents, rather than smoothly distended as with a primary impaction.

SMALL INTESTINAL DISTENSION

Distension of the small intestine may be palpable in grass disease, enteritis, strangulation obstruction, impaction, intussusception and non-strangulating infarction. The number of loops palpable depends on the nature, the duration and the location of the lesion. In severe cases involving the more distal jejunum or ileum, multiple loops are palpable within the abdomen and may extend back to the pelvic cavity. The loops are recognized by their diameter (often 5–10 cm) and the lack of taenial bands.

Occasionally, small intestinal intussusception can be diagnosed per rectum. The gut involved has a thickened, rubbery feel and the limits of the intussuscepted portion may be palpable. However, the major rectal finding is often related to the obstructing effect of the intussusception in producing distension of the more proximal jejunum, i.e. loops of distended small intestine. The intussusception may be limited to the small intestine but ileocaecal intussusceptions also occur.

The most common site of small intestinal impaction is the ileum. If rectal examination is undertaken during the early stages of the disease, the impacted ileum is palpable medial to the caecum. In later hours this is not so as the jejunum fills with gas and fluid and these loops obscure the ileum. Surgery is required as medical therapy tends to be ineffective in cleaning the impaction.

Anterior enteritis or gastroduodenitis produces characteristic rectal findings. There is distension of the duodenum and this can be discerned as the intestine passes caudal to the root of the mesentery, across the caudal aspect of the caecum.

If an ileal obstruction is present and, especially if this involves strangulation, there is often a marked pain response to pulling of the medial caecal taenia in a caudal direction.

CAECAL INTUSSUSCEPTION

Invagination of the caecal apex resulting in a caecocaecal intussusception is a well recognized entity. On rectal examination, a mass can be palpated within the caecum. The ileocaecal region may be affected producing some small intestinal distension.

LARGE INTESTINAL GASEOUS DISTENSION

This occurs in a number of conditions including primary flatulent colic, transverse or small colon obstruction (e.g. enteroliths or pedunculated lipomas), large colon displacements and large colon torsions. The degree of distension varies but the abnormal viscus may be palpable at the pelvic inlet or within the pelvis; this is usually the case with torsions of 360° or more. Gross abdominal distension is generally present.

It may be possible with experience to determine the exact nature of the torsion or displacement such as right dorsal displacement of the colon. However, surgical treatment may be presumed to be necessary with gross distension and, or, persistent presence of abnormally tight and painful taenial bands. An additional helpful factor in identification of positional abnormalities which have affected the vascular supply and drainage is oedema of the gut wall, and especially of the mesocolon. If this is present in cases with persistent colic but no great distension, a partial torsion of the colon should be suspected.

ENTRAPMENT OF LARGE COLON

Entrapment occurs when the left large colon migrates dorsally between the spleen and the body wall and then passes medial to the spleen, coming to lie over the nephrosplenic ligament. It is known also as left dorsal displacement of the colon. Very occasionally small intestine or small colon can be trapped similarly. Rectal findings depend upon the location of the entrapment along the length of the colon and upon whether or not blockage of the gut results.

In mild cases, no secondary impaction or distension is

present but the colon can be palpated as it is fixed in the cranial dorsal left quadrant of the abdomen and from there runs in a dorsoventral direction. It may be possible to palpate the nephrosplenic ligament and to ascertain that some gut lies dorsal to it. In other cases secondary impaction or gaseous distension of the left colon is present; these range from mild to severe. Severe gaseous distension does not permit examination of the cranial abdomen but it may be possible to determine that the distended gut is passing towards the nephrosplenic region in more moderate cases.

PERITONITIS

The normal peritoneum is non-painful and smooth. Peritonitis may lead to an adverse response to rectal examination due to pain and it may be possible to detect some roughening of parietal or visceral peritoneum or adhesions between perito-neal surfaces. If gut rupture has occurred, especially of the colon, gut contents are often palpable on the serosa of the intestine. Also a pneumoperitoneum may be present. This is characterized by moderate abdominal distension but only mild to moderate gut distension and an ease of movement in the abdomen during rectal examination.

SMALL INTESTINAL MUSCULAR HYPERTROPHY

This occurs in response to a slowly developing occlusive lesion and may result in recurrent, or more rarely, acute colic. The most common location is the ileum (e.g. ileocaecal valve abnormalities, ileo-ileal intussusceptions, ileal lymphosar-comata) but jejunal cases have been recorded also. Secondary hypertrophy of several metres of intestine may be present and, if palpable, presents as a length of thickened gut with a hose-pipe rigidity. This can be differentiated from gut which is contracting and may therefore feel thickened transiently as with hypertrophy there is no alteration in diameter or texture over a period of time.

INTRA-ABDOMINAL ABSCESS FORMATION OR NEOPLASIA

In these cases the mass(es) may be palpable per rectum if they are situated in a suitable position. There may be one or more large abscesses or tumours (possibly giving rise to weight loss or colic) or there may be discernible increases in the lymphoid tissue. This is palpable particularly in the mesocolon of the large colon and the presence of multiple nodules may indicate an infective, an inflammatory or a neoplastic condition.

SIGNIFICANCE OF RECTAL FINDINGS

No one part of a clinical examination should be carried out in isolation and therefore any abnormalities suspected by rectal palpation should be considered in the light of the general clinical assessment. However, in many cases, the rectal findings are crucial to any decision for surgery. Other diagnostic aids should be used (see below), especially if an anterior obstruction is suspected.

The presence of distended loops of small intestine indicates the need for surgery unless the distension is not great, the gut sounds are hyperactive and there is a marked pyrexia ($> 40°C$) in which case salmonellosis or another form of enteritis may be present. Small intestinal impaction, large colon displacements or torsions and small colon obstructions also require surgical intervention. It may be necessary to perform rectal examinations at hourly or two hourly intervals if the case is seen close to the onset of colic. This can be useful especially in cases where some increased tautness of the large intestinal taenial bands can be felt but with no associated colonic distension. This tautness could be due to gut contractions and is not necessarily pathological. However, if their presence persists over a number of hours and there is still evidence of pain, a displacement should be suspected. Alternatively, if there is a distal small intestinal obstruction, distended intestine may not be palpable on the initial examination but becomes apparent as the condition progresses.

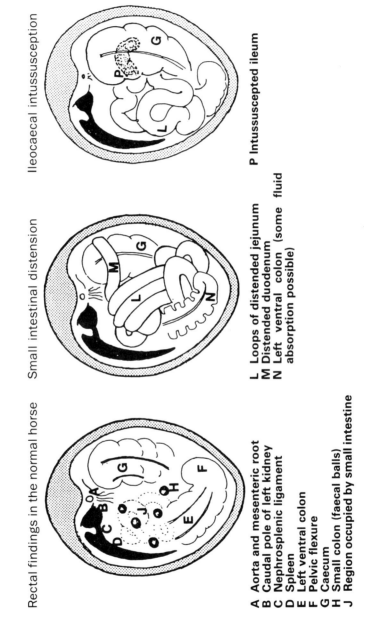

Rectal findings in the normal horse   Small intestinal distension   Ileocaecal intussusception

A Aorta and mesenteric root
B Caudal pole of left kidney
C Nephrosplenic ligament
D Spleen
E Left ventral colon
F Pelvic flexure
G Caecum
H Small colon (faecal balls)
J Region occupied by small intestine

L Loops of distended jejunum
M Distended duodenum
N Left ventral colon (some fluid absorption possible)

P Intussuscepted ileum

Fig. 8.1 Rectal findings in the normal horse and in some specific pathological conditions. Figures after Kopf (1982) *Proc. Int. Symp. Colic Res.* **1**, 236–260.

Ileal impaction

Caecal intussusception

Large colon torsion

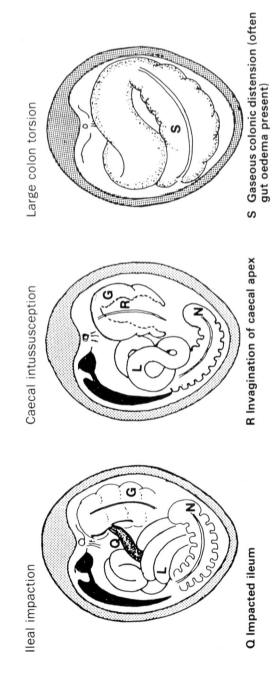

Q Impacted ileum

R Invagination of caecal apex

S Gaseous colonic distension (often gut oedema present)

Fig. 8.1 *Cont.*

Right dorsal displacement of large colon

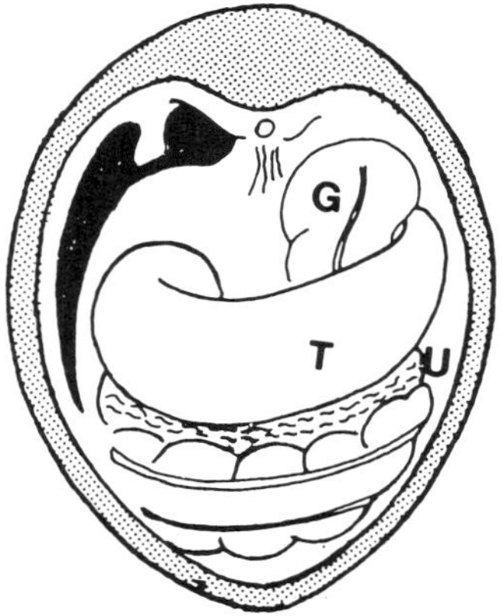

Nephrosplenic entrapment of the large colon

Nephrosplenic entrapment of the large colon

T Colon displaced to right, lateral to caecum
U Oedematous mesocolon

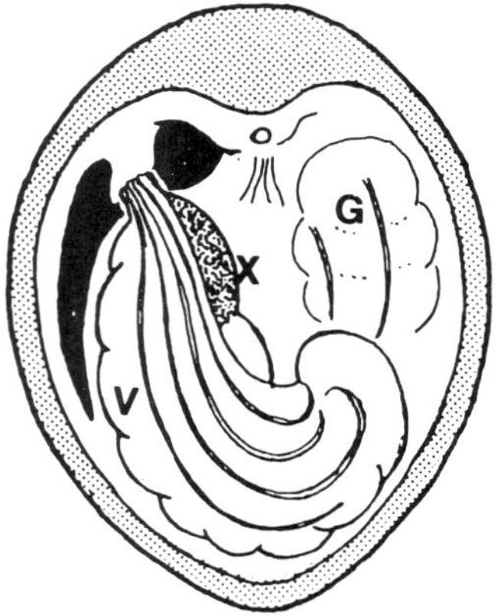

V Majority of the large colon cascading down from the nephrosplenic region
X Moderate impaction of the left dorsal colon

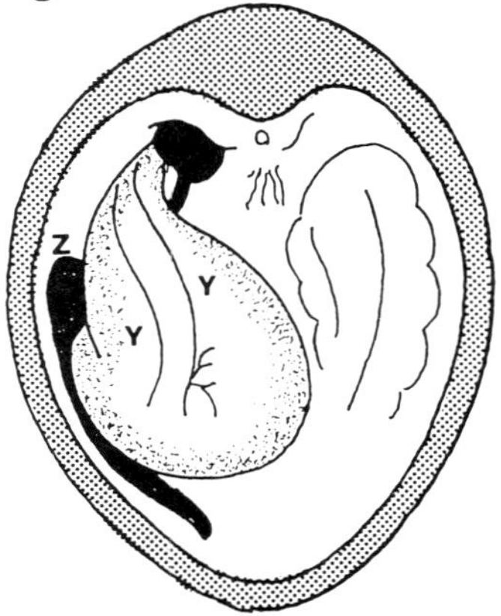

Y Impacted left ventral and dorsal colon by entrapment at the junction of right and left colon
Z Ventromedial displacement of the spleen

Fig. 8.1 *Cont.*

ADDITIONAL DIAGNOSTIC TECHNIQUES

Nasogastric intubation

In cases with gastric distension this can be vital to survival in addition to aiding diagnosis. The horse rarely vomits (material is voided through the nose rather than the mouth) and gastric rupture is a more probable sequel to severe distension. It is important to realize that it may require persistence (3–5 min) in applying suction (by mouth) and in altering the position of the tube before the sequestrated fluid is obtained. Nothing should be given by stomach tube unless a specific diagnosis has been made (e.g. liquid paraffin for pelvic flexure impaction) and until suction has been applied and no reflux has been obtained.

Reflux of more than 2 litres of fluid indicates gastric retention, e.g. grass disease, small intestine obstruction and, or, gastroduodenitis.

Contrast radiography

With the exceptions of oesophageal studies and gastroduodenal obstructions in foals, radiography does not aid diagnosis of gut disorders.

Paracentesis abdominis

Collection of peritoneal fluid is a useful and simple technique. It does not require sophisticated equipment and provides useful information even with visual inspection rather than laboratory assessment. The ventral midline caudal to the sternum should be clipped and scrubbed as for surgery. A 2 in needle (19 or 21 gauge) is necessary in most animals because of the depth of retroperitoneal fat. The needle should be inserted in the midline at 90° to the long axis of the body. If no fluid is obtained, the needle should be rotated to encourage flow; if this is unsuccessful the procedure may be repeated at two other points along the midline (3–4 cm apart).

Interpretation of peritoneal fluid abnormalities is based on the understanding that the fluid reflects changes in the peritoneum itself. Normal fluid is clear and straw coloured; peritonitis causes an increase in leucocytes and the fluid becomes more turbid and grey-white. Gut infarction produces an increase in both leucocytes and erythrocytes and thus the fluid becomes sanguinous and turbid. Torsion of the large colon produces mucosal ischaemia before that of the serosa and therefore lack of blood stained peritoneal fluid does not rule out this condition.

If the first few drops appear blood tinged but this then clears, blood vessel puncture should be suspected and a fresh sample pot used to collect the later fluid for assessment. In some cases of gut entrapment over the nephrosplenic ligament, blood is obtained by paracentesis as the spleen comes to lie in the ventral midline and may be punctured during the procedure. The presence of gut contents (green or brown tinged and particulate matter) may indicate gut rupture or could be due to enterocentesis. Other factors such as any sudden deterioration, sweating, muscle tremors, pulse rate and character, the presence or absence of haemoconcentration and rectal findings must be used to attempt differentiation of these two possibilities.

Ultrasound

This may be helpful to confirm the presence of intra-abdominal masses but is not useful in acute colic cases.

RECTAL RUPTURE

The possibility of rectal rupture is present during each rectal examination. With proper care and if necessary, sedation, the likelihood is extremely low and should not deter veterinary surgeons from performing such examinations.

An injury can be graded as follows:

Grade I   Mucosal/submucosal involvement
Grade II   Muscle involvement
Grade III   Tearing of all layers except the serosa
Grade IV   Complete perforation

The most common site is at the level of the pelvic inlet in

the dorsal wall of the rectum. It may be caudal to the peritoneal reflexion and the mesentery may have a limiting effect on contamination. The condition should be suspected if there is a feeling of "give" during the examination, if there is blood on the hand or arm and, or, if there is persistent straining following examination.

Immediate therapy includes sedation and, or, epidural analgesia, broad spectrum antibiotic therapy, tetanus antitoxin administration and possibly atropine to decrease gut propulsion (0·1 mg/kg intravenously). Assessment by a speculum or gentle manual palpation should be performed if a grade III or IV lesion is suspected but must be done under an epidural block or general anaesthesia. The prognosis with a grade I or II injury is good with a laxative diet and no further rectal interference for at least 6 weeks. Grade III lesions may heal with similar management but carry a worse prognosis. Complete rupture requires a colostomy or the insertion of a liner tube and has a guarded prognosis. The warning signs should not be ignored or treatment delayed as the prognosis decreases with such delay.

CONCLUSION

Rectal examination should form part of a complete clinical assessment of equine gastrointestinal disorders. Some appreciation of the normal anatomic configuration aids detection and interpretation of pathological findings. However, many colic cases do not require great experience before such interpretation becomes feasible. It may not be possible to be absolutely specific but the indication for medical or surgical treatment can be gained. Common abnormalities include gut distension (due to gas, fluid or ingesta), gut spasm, gut displacement, painful areas and lack of rectal faeces together with dryness of the rectal mucosa.

ACKNOWLEDGEMENTS

The author wishes to thank Professor G. B. Edwards for the illustrations and Mrs A. Harris for typing the manuscript.

CHAPTER 9

Auriculopalpebral and Palpebral Nerve Blocks

PETER BEDFORD

INTRODUCTION

Forceful closure of the palpebral fissure during examination or resulting from blepharospasm renders evaluation of the globe and intraocular structures impossible in the horse. The

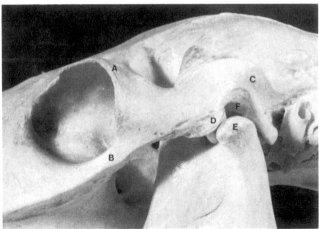

Fig. 9.1 Identification of bones. A, supraorbital process of the frontal bone; B, zygomatic process of the malar bone; C, zygomatic process of the squamous temporal bone; D, condyle of the squamous temporal bone; E, condyle of the mandible; F, glenoid cavity of the squamous temporal bone.

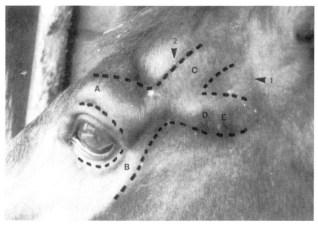

Fig. 9.2
Position of nerve blocks. A–E, see Fig. 9.1; 1, auriculopalpebral block; 2, palpebral block.

eyelid sphincter muscle, orbicularis oculi, is powerful in this species, and digital force alone is insufficient to allow a thorough examination. Corneal and conjunctival pain may be controlled by a topical analgesic, but difficulty may again be experienced in parting the lids to allow its application.

REGIONAL ANALGESIA

Regional analgesia can be obtained by blocking the frontal nerve at the level of the supraorbital foramen, while the zygomatic nerve can be blocked along the ventral rim of the orbit. The lacrimal nerve is located along the dorsal rim of the orbit just medial to the lateral canthus. This may allow minor surgery to be completed and can be used to supplement auriculopalpebral and palpebral nerve blocks.

AURICULOPALPEBRAL AND PALPEBRAL NERVE BLOCK

Akinesia of the eyelids is easily achieved in the horse by blocking the facial supply to the orbicularis oculi muscle at the level of either the auriculopalpebral nerve or its palpebral branch. The auriculopalpebral nerve arises deep to the parotid gland and the superficial temporal artery, its auricular branch passing dorsally to innervate the anterior auricular and par-otido-auricularis muscles and its palpebral (temporal) branch passing anteriorly and obliquely over the zygomatic process of the squamous temporal bone and then forwards towards the upper eyelid in the subcutaneous tissue along the dorsomedial edge of the arch. (The relevant bones are identified in Figure 9.1). Further division of the palpebral nerve anterior to the supraorbital process of the frontal bone allows innervation of both the upper and lower eyelids. Blocking the auriculopalpeb-ral nerve or its palpebral branch can render the eyelids relatively immobile during examination and of the two blocks perhaps the latter is the easier to achieve. The site is easier to define as the dorsal edge of the zygomatic arch is a readily palpable structure.

TECHNIQUE

The use of a twitch or even sedation may be necessary to complete the block. The auriculopalpebral nerve is reached by infiltrating local analgesic into the depression found ventral to the temporal part of the zygomatic arch just posterior to the ramus of the mandible. The needle should be directed towards the highest point on the dorsal edge of the zygomatic arch, and approximately 7 or 8 ml of the analgesic injected into the area. Alternatively the palpebral branch of the nerve can be blocked by injecting a similar amount of the analgesic just medial to the highest point of the zygomatic arch (Fig. 9.2). Following successful block the membrana nictitans tends to protrude, there is ptosis and the palpebral fissure narrows.

CHAPTER 10

Nasolacrimal Cannulation

SHEILA CRISPIN

INTRODUCTION

The basic components of the nasolacrimal drainage apparatus can be delineated by dacryocystorhinography (Figs 10.1 and 10.2). Five to 10 ml of contrast medium (meglumine iothalamate, Conray 280; RMB) can be injected via the lacrimal puncta, or retrograde through the nasal ostium.

The nasolacrimal duct is contained within a bony canal during its passage through the lacrimal bone, but more rostrally, as it passes via the lacrimal groove of the maxilla, it is covered at first by cartilage and then by the mucous membrane of the middle meatus. The terminal part of the duct lies in the ventral nasal conchal fold and opens on the skin of the floor of the nostril, close to the mucocutaneous junction. The nasal ostium (Fig. 10.3) is readily visualized in horses so that investigations of the nasolacrimal drainage apparatus in this species usually commence rostrally.

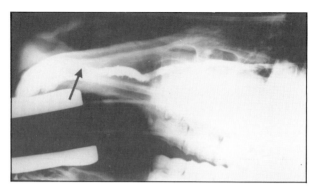

Fig. 10.1 Lateral dacryocystorhinogram of a horse. The upper punctum has been cannulated, the lower punctum occluded. Contrast medium (Conray 280) delineates the nasolacrimal drainage apparatus. The presumptive site of the nasal ostium is indicated by a closed arrow but no contrast medium extends beyond this point because of congenital atresia.

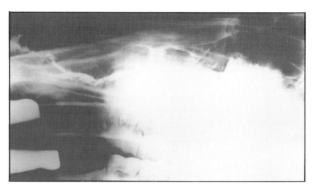

Fig. 10.2 Lateral dacryocystorhinogram of the same horse as that shown in Fig. 10.1. The nasal ostium has been surgically created and contrast medium now passes freely through the drainage apparatus.

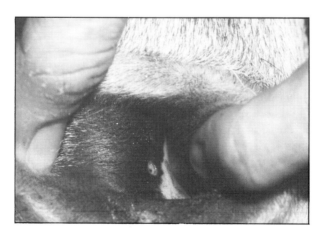

Fig. 10.3
External nares of horse folded back to show the nasal ostium.

CANNULATION

The importance of investigating all aspects of tear secretion and drainage in the evaluation of the nasolacrimal drainage apparatus has been emphasized previously; in horses, cannulation and catheterization of the nasolacrimal drainage apparatus are used for the assessment and retention of patency and as a means of delivering therapeutic agents to the eye.

TECHNIQUE

For cannulation of the nasal ostium topical local analgesic, for example, proxymetacaine hydrochloride drops (Ophthaine; Ciba-Geigy), lignocaine hydrochloride gel or ointment (Xylocaine; Astra), applied to this region a few minutes before cannulation is usually adequate in tractable animals. In more difficult patients a twitch is applied to the lower lip and, or, chemical sedation with an agent like detomidine hydrochloride (Domosedan; Smith Kline) is employed.

The cannula, or catheter, is usually introduced a centimetre or so into the lacrimal duct (Fig. 10.4) and 5–10 ml of sterile saline injected in retrograde fashion by applying moderate pressure to the syringe. In some horses it may help subsequent investigations if a small quantity of local analgesic

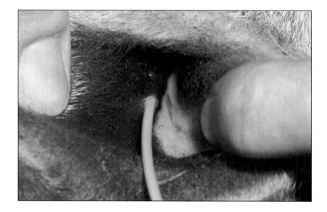

Fig. 10.4
External nares of a horse to show a catheter inserted into the nasolacrimal drainage apparatus via the nasal ostium.

(proxymetacaine hydrochloride) is injected initially, with other irrigating fluids following several minutes later. If the system is patent saline should flow from the lacrimal puncta near the medial canthus; the possibility of nervous patients reacting unfavourably to the procedure should be borne in mind. Retrograde irrigation will differentiate partial or complete impatency of the nasolacrimal duct of either, or both, canaliculi. This technique is also valuable if therapeutic agents are to be applied to the eye. A commercially available indwelling cannula (Portex; Arnolds Veterinary Products) (Fig. 10.5) can be sutured in place when frequent or prolonged treatment is required and offers a useful alternative to subpalpebral delivery systems.

On occasions it may be necessary to cannulate the nasolacrimal drainage apparatus via the puncta, particularly if material is required for culture, or when surgery is to be performed in this area (Fig. 10.6). In the conscious animal sedation may be required and topical analgesia is desirable. The upper punctum is usually cannulated (Fig. 10.7), but the lower punctum can also be used. Monofilament nylon (1–3) can be used to probe

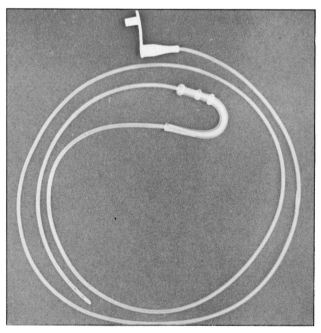

Fig. 10.5
Indwelling nasolacrimal cannula. (Portex; Arnolds Veterinary Products) designed for use in horses.

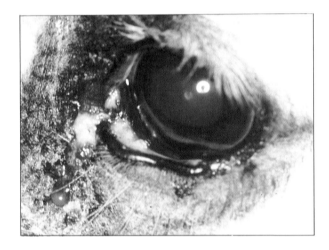

Fig. 10.6
Adult horse with a
neoplasm (equine
sarcoid) which has
obstructed the lower
punctum of the left
eye. The upper
punctum was patent.

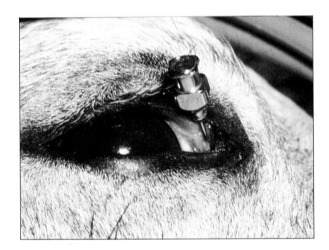

Fig. 10.7
Adult horse with a
nasolacrimal cannula
inserted into the
upper punctum.

the nasolacrimal drainage system although the end should be heated in a flame to blunt it so as to prevent trauma. The nylon can be used on its own or as a guide for subsequent passage of a catheter. Usually, however, a suitably sized cannula (Portex; Arnolds Veterinary Products) or urinary catheter (FG 6–10) is inserted and a 10 ml syringe attached. Gentle but firm irrigation may demonstrate patency or, for example, in animals with distal (rostral) atresia (Fig. 10.8) a fluctuating bulge may be noted at the presumptive site of the nasal ostium. Surgical creation of the nasal ostium is a relatively straightforward procedure which will correct the defect, although it may be necessary to suture a catheter in place within the nasolacrimal drainage apparatus to retain patency once the surgery has been completed. For surgery which involves the canaliculi a short length of polythene tubing (external diameter 2–3 mm) is used and this is usually removed 5–10 days after surgery (Figs. 10.9–10.11). Patency of the nasolacrimal drainage apparatus can be confirmed by instilling fluorescein dye (Minims; SNP) into the conjunctival sac (Fig. 10.12).

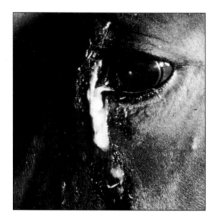

Fig. 10.8
Foal with congenital atresia of the nasal ostium showing the considerable discharge which accompanies this condition.

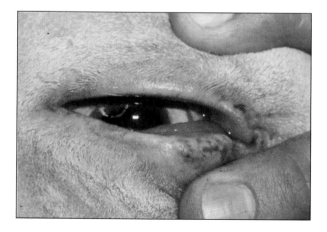

Fig. 10.9
Adult horse with large, reasonably well circumscribed, neoplasm of the lower eyelid (carcinoma) which involved the lower lacrimal canaliculus.

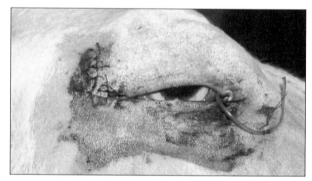

Fig. 10.10 The same animal as shown above immediately after surgery. The lower punctum was catheterized before surgery and the catheter was sutured in place. The tumour was completely excised and the catheter was removed five days after surgery once the patency of the canaliculus was assured. The blepharoplastic procedure used for this case is as described by J.S.A. Spreull (1982). *The Veterinary Annual*, 22nd Issue, pp.279–297. John Wright and Sons.

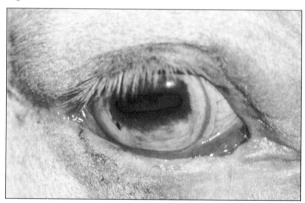

Fig. 10.11
The same animal just over a month after surgery.

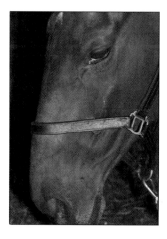

Fig. 10.12
Fluorescein dye used to demonstrate patency of the nasolacrimal drainage apparatus.

ACKNOWLEDGEMENTS

I am grateful to Dr C. Gibbs for allowing me to publish dacryocystorhinograms from the horse and to Mr J. J. Yeats, the surgeon responsible for the equine case shown in Figs. 10.1 and 10.2. I am also grateful to Mr S. J. Butterworth for allowing me to publish details of one of his equine cases illustrated in Figs. 10.9, 10.10 and 10.11. Some of the photographic material was kindly supplied by Mr J. Conibear and Mr M. Parsons. Many thanks to Mrs V. Beswetherick, Mrs C. Francis and Mrs M. Hughes for typing the manuscript.

CHAPTER 11

Clinical Aspects of Equine Cardiology

BRENDAN GLAZIER

INTRODUCTION

Examination of the heart is an essential part of a general examination in the horse, whether before sale or for insurance. It should always be carried out before the administration of an anaesthetic or tranquillizing agent. Even well-tried drugs may, on rare occasions, produce fatal side effects. In these circumstances, if a heart examination was not carried out before the drug was administered, a charge of negligence might be levied against the veterinarian.

Most heart conditions can either be detected or suspected from a simple stethoscope examination. Whether one examines horses regularly or occasionally, it is prudent to carry out the examination systematically. In this way obvious conditions or signs will not be missed.

A comprehensive history should be obtained. The physical examination should include a general inspection of the animal followed by palpation of the arterial pulse, chest wall and sternum. This should be followed by auscultation of the heart.

GENERAL EXAMINATION

Note the animal's stance and physical condition at rest in the box. Poor condition is frequently a prominent sign of endocarditis. Note the respiratory rate and pattern. Respiratory distress may be associated with acute mitral insufficiency or, in young foals or yearlings, with congenital heart disease.

Observe the condition of the jugular vein on both sides of the neck when the head is in the normal erect position. Normally pulsations are seen in the lower region of the veins near the entrance to the chest. Abnormal prominent pulsations extending a variable distance up the vein in the neck may be associated with an incompetent tricuspid valve arising from endocarditis or from dilatation of the valvular ring because of marked enlargement of the right ventricle.

Distension (cording) of the jugular vein may occur without abnormal pulsations in right-sided heart failure, in pericarditis with effusion, in constrictive pericarditis, and with calcification of the vessels following the administration of excessive amounts of vitamin D in foals and yearlings.

A distended pulseless jugular vein may be observed when the vein is thrombosed or the blood flow in the anterior vena cava is obstructed.

The cardiac impulse can be seen in a zone around the point of the elbow on the left thoracic wall. It is not normally seen on the right thoracic wall.

Oedema, either confined to the sternum or extending backwards along the abdominal wall and sometimes extending into the limbs, may be seen in right-sided heart failure.

The mucous membranes should be pink and the capillary refill time about 2 s. Cyanosis of mucous membranes is not a common finding in heart disease in the horse. It may occur with left heart failure and in congenital cardiac defects where there is significant mixing of venous with arterial blood (right to left shunts).

PALPATION

The jugular veins should be palpated to detect distensions which may be masked by a long coat. Similarly, a search should be made for oedema in the dependent parts.

The arterial pulse may be palpated at a number of sites: the transverse facial arterial site, the mandibular artery, the carotid and digital arteries. The pulse is weak and thready in shock and in heart failure involving the left ventricle. It is bounding in cases of marked aortic incompetence and in long-standing cases of ductus arteriosus. The pulse may be single or double; a double pulse may be detected in association with pure aortic incompetence or pure aortic stenosis. It should be noted, however, that a dicrotic pulse, i.e. a double pulse where the amplitude of the first of the pair is higher than the second, occurs normally in the horse when the heart is beating slowly.

AUSCULTATION OF THE HEART

Auscultation is one of the most important parts of the cardiac examination. Both sides of the chest should be auscultated using both the bell and the diaphragm chest pieces of the stethoscope in turn. The bell chest piece accentuates low frequency sounds while the diaphragm accentuates high frequencies. Auscultation should be carried out over as wide an area as possible; the chest piece should be "inched" around the chest, rather than concentrating on a few specific areas.

There are five auscultatory areas where the sounds produced at various valves are best relayed (Fig. 11.1). For a horse in a normal standing posture with both forelimbs equally loaded, not one in front of the other, the areas are:

Mitral area: This is on the left thoracic wall at a level midway between a horizontal line drawn through the point of the shoulder and the sternum, at the caudal edge of the triceps muscle (fifth intercostal space).

Aortic area: Found on the left thoracic wall, about 3 cm below the level of a horizontal line through the point of the shoulder at the edge of, and extending slightly cranially under, the triceps.

Pulmonary area: This is situated on the left thoracic wall slightly below the level of the aortic area and about 3 cm in front of the aortic area under the triceps (third intercostal space). Pulling the left forelimb forward may facilitate listening at this area.

Apex: The apex is on the left thoracic wall in the region of the point of the elbow. From here it extends cranially and caudally for 3–4 cm.

Tricuspid area: This is on the right thoracic wall under the edge of the triceps. Sounds associated with the right ventricle are best heard here but they may also be detected on the left thoracic wall in an area situated cranially to the pulmonary area, situated deeply under the triceps.

HEART SOUNDS

Heart sounds are audible vibrations resulting from acceleration or deceleration in the flow of blood. All four sounds may be heard in normal horses during an examination. In most horses, however, only three sounds may be heard, either S4, S1 and S2 or S1, S2 and S3. In some normal horses only S1 and S2 are audible.

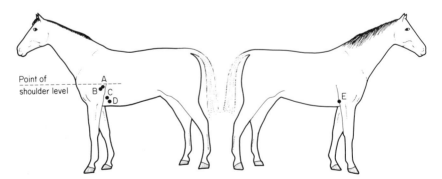

Fig. 11.1 Auscultatory areas. The apex, the mitral, aortic and pulmonary areas are situated on the left thoracic wall. The tricuspid area is on the right thoracic wall. A, Aortic; B, Pulmonary; C, Mitral; D, Apex; E, Tricuspid.

CAUSES OF HEART SOUNDS

Only the major event associated with the production of each sound is given.

First heart sound

The first heart sound (S1) often referred to as the "lubb" sound is associated with closure of the atrioventricular (mitral and tricuspid) valves at the beginning of contraction (systole) of the ventricles. It is best heard at the apex on the left thoracic wall. It coincides with the apex beat on the chest wall. S1 is usually longer, louder and of a lower pitch than S2.

The intensity of S1 increases directly with the speed and the distance the cusps of the atrioventricular valves travel in closing. With the increased heart rate of exercise, fear or excitement, S1 is loud because the a-v valve cusps are widely separated when the ventricles begin to contract and the increased force of the heart beat causes them to shut rapidly.

The intensity of S1, and that of the other sounds, may be decreased owing to damping of sound by excessive muscular development on the chest wall, obesity, dense coat or excess fluid in the thorax or pericardial sac.

A beat-to-beat variation in the intensity of S1 may occur with atrioventricular heart block, atrial fibrillation, premature beats and with ventricular tachycardia.

Splitting of S1 may occur when there is significant asynchrony in the contractions of the right and left ventricles, as in premature beats or bundle branch block. Since splitting of the first heart sound may occur in the normal equine heart it is not a reliable sign of heart disease in the horse.

Second heart sound

The second heart sound (S2) is also referred to as the "dup" sound. It occurs at the beginning of relaxation of the ventricles and is associated with closure of the semilunar (aortic and pulmonary) valves. S2 is best heard near the base of the heart over the aortic and pulmonary auscultatory area on the left thoracic wall. Splitting of S2 may occur in normal horses, those with severe chronic obstructive pulmonary disease, and with atrial septal defect.

The third heart sound frequently follows S2 and should not be confused with a splitting or doubling of S2. In some pulmonary disorders S2 may be particularly loud.

Third heart sound

The third heart sound (S3) is associated with the rapid ventricular filling phase of the ventricles. It is frequently heard in normal horses. It is best heard at the apex or mitral area on the left thoracic wall.

In the normal horse the intensity of S3 may vary and it may disappear with a change in heart rate. The intensity of S3 may increase in congestive heart failure, constrictive pericarditis and in mitral incompetence. On its own, a loud S3 is not a reliable sign of cardiac disease; other signs should be sought.

Fourth heart sound

The fourth heart sound (S4) frequently referred to as the atrial sound, is associated with contraction of the atria. It occurs just before S1; it is best heard in the mitral area, when the resting heart rate is low. When dropped beats occur in second degree atrioventricular heart block, S4 may be heard as an isolated sound near the beginning of the pauses. The sound is likened to that produced when a finger is quickly stroked across the palm of one's hand.

The presence of S4 denotes that an organized atrial contraction has occurred. The presence of S4 helps to differentiate innocuous a-v heart block from atrial fibrillation, because it occurs in the former but not in the latter.

CLICKS

In normal horses a click may be heard between S1 and S2, usually in mid-interval. Clicks are usually best heard on the left thoracic wall, either at the heart base or over the mitral area. The cause has not been determined and in the horse, clicks are generally considered to be benign. In man, clicks are common, being frequently associated with prolapse of the mitral valve into the left atrium.

In one horse a transient, remarkably loud, clicking sound was heard immediately after exercise. The sound resembled that of a ticking clock and could be heard when standing close to the animal. This horse also had atrial fibrillation.

MURMURS

Murmurs have a longer duration than heart sounds and are audible during normally silent intervals in the cardiac cycle. It is generally accepted that while heart sounds are caused by sudden alterations in the speed of the blood flow, murmurs are caused by turbulence or vortices in the flow.

While murmurs are classified according to their intensity, it should be noted that the intensity of a murmur may not be a reliable guide to the extent of the lesion. Relatively small lesions may have loud murmurs and extensive lesions low intensity murmurs. Much knowledge regarding murmurs is empirical.

Murmurs may be cardiac or extracardiac in origin. Those associated with organic heart disease are referred to as organic (pathological) murmurs (Table 11.1) while those which occur in the absence of organic heart disease are referred to as functional (non-pathological) murmurs (Table 11.2). If it is difficult to decide whether a murmur is organic or not, the decision may have to be postponed for 2–3 months. It is not uncommon to find that, for no obvious reasons, some loud murmurs disappear after a period of 6 weeks.

CLASSIFICATION OF MURMURS

Timing

A murmur may occur at any place in the cardiac cycle (Fig. 11.2).

Table 11.1 Pathological murmurs.

All murmurs accompanied by a thrill.

Pansystolic (regurgitant) murmurs; include those
of mitral incompetence, tricuspid incompetence,
and ventricular septal defect.

All prolonged diastolic murmurs; includes those of
aortic valve incompetence, or less commonly
pulmonary valve incompetence.

A continuous murmur in subjects older than 4
days old.

Table 11.2 Non-pathological murmurs.

Grade 1/6 and 2/6 systolic murmurs.
Murmurs that disappear on exercise.
Murmurs that are intermittent.
Murmurs that arise from anaemia.
Continuous murmur of patent ductus arteriosus in
foals up to 4 days old; if heard beyond this it is
usually abnormal.
Grade 3/6 systolic murmur near the base of the
heart in foals up to 4 days old.
Cardiorespiratory murmur. Caused by heart
pumping air in the lung.
Faint, short, blowing diastolic murmur shortly
after the second heart sound.
"Two-year-old squeak". Short musical diastolic
murmur resembling a faint whistle, squeak or
coo.

It should be clearly understood that this category
includes only murmurs that occur in the absence of
other signs of cardiovascular disease.

Systolic murmurs

These occur during contraction of the ventricles (systole),
between S1 and S2. There are three main types of systolic
murmur: pansystolic, holosystolic and merosystolic. A pansystolic murmur begins with S1 and extends right into S2.
A holosystolic murmur extends from S1 to S2 but does not

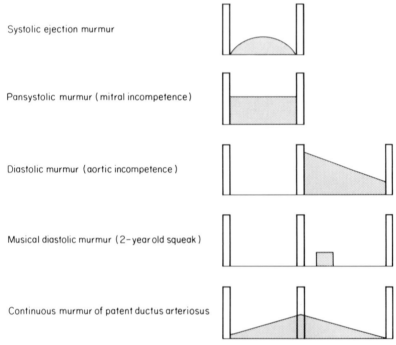

Systolic ejection murmur

Pansystolic murmur (mitral incompetence)

Diastolic murmur (aortic incompetence)

Musical diastolic murmur (2-year old squeak)

Continuous murmur of patent ductus arteriosus

Fig. 11.2 Diagrammatic representation of common systolic and diastolic murmurs.

encroach on either sound. Merosystolic murmurs occupy only a part of the systolic interval but finish well before S2.

A systolic murmur which ends before S2 may be referred to as an ejection murmur; one that does not end before S2 may be referred to as a systolic regurgitant murmur.

In horses, ejection murmurs are common. They are best heard at the base of the heart in the aortic and pulmonary areas; they peak early and are crescendo–decrescendo or decrescendo in shape. These murmurs are generally believed to be associated with increased blood flow at the outflow tracts at the ventricles or in the large vessels just beyond them. They are usually non-pathological.

Transitory murmurs may develop with excitement or exercise in some apparently normal horses and are considered to be flow related and non-pathological.

Not infrequently, a grade 3/6 systolic murmur (ejection murmur) can be heard on the right thoracic wall in the tricuspid area. This murmur is believed to be associated with non-laminar flow in the aorta or incompetence of the tricuspid valve. In the absence of a thrill, abnormal jugular pulsations and abnormal arterial pulsations some horses appear to compensate and race well. Care must be exercised to avoid this type of murmur being confused with that of a ventricular septal defect which is heard on both sides of the chest and is usually accompanied by a thrill.

Systolic murmurs may also develop during the course of severe anaemia or during colic; they usually disappear when the condition is corrected.

Diastolic murmurs

Diastolic murmurs occur during diastole, between S2 of one beat and S1 of the next. Most of them occur either early or late in diastole while others span the entire length of diastole. They may be divided into two types: regurgitant murmurs, arising from an incompetent (leaking) aortic or pulmonary valve, and murmurs associated with filling of the ventricles.

Regurgitant diastolic murmurs are relatively common in older horses, especially aged stallions. They are long and usually occur because of incompetence of the aortic valve; pure incompetence of the pulmonary valve is rare in the horse.

Functional diastolic murmurs are rather common in the equine heart, occurring early or late in diastole, and are usually short. The most easily identifiable functional (ventricular filling) murmur is the "2-year-old squeak". This murmur is common in 2-year-olds but may also occur in younger and in much older horses. It is usually best heard in the mitral area although it may also be heard in the aortic and tricuspid area. It may be constant or intermittent, occurs shortly after S2 and resembles a whistle, a squeak or a cooing sound.

Another innocuous early diastolic murmur is a short blowing one which occurs shortly after S2 and, like the "2-year-old squeak", it may be constant or intermittent and is perhaps a variant of this murmur.

A functional diastolic murmur may also be heard late in diastole, beginning just before S1. It is low-pitched, rumbling and brief.

Continuous murmur

Here the murmur continues from S1 of one beat to S1 of the next; it occurs throughout the cardiac cycle. The most common cause is a patent ductus arteriosus in the newborn foal. The murmur develops because of the production of a high velocity jet of blood travelling from the high pressure aorta to the low pressure pulmonary artery through the patent ductus arteriosus. When the ductus arteriosus closes, the murmur disappears. It should disappear in the normal foal within 4 days.

In severe anaemia, a continuous murmur, referred to as a venous hum, may be detected by auscultating over the jugular veins at the entrance to the chest. From here it may be relayed to the chest wall. The murmur, however, can be temporarily abolished by manually occluding the jugular veins.

Intensity of murmurs

A scale of six arbitrary grades is recommended (Table 11.3). In this scale, murmurs with an intensity of 4/6 or more are considered to be pathological under most circumstances.

Site of maximum intensity and radiation

An effort should be made to locate the site of maximum intensity of the murmur in relation to the auscultatory areas. This helps to locate the site of origin of the murmur. The radiation of a murmur may provide clues as to its origin. Aortic murmurs are best heard at the base of the heart and may radiate for a variable distance into the neck, along the jugular furrow, sometimes almost to the base of the ear. The continuous murmur of patent ductus arteriosus is best heard at the base of the heart, in the pulmonary and aortic areas. In ventricular septal defect (the most common congenital defect in the equine heart) the murmur is most intense in an area low down on the right thoracic wall. The systolic murmur of pulmonary stenosis is loudest at the base of the heart, in the pulmonic area. The systolic murmur of mitral incompetence may best be heard in the mitral area and may radiate towards the base of the heart.

Table 11.3 Grading of murmurs 1-6 system

1/6	Nearly imperceptible murmur confined to a small area on the chest wall.
2/6	Faint murmur clearly audible after a few seconds auscultation.
3/6	Murmur readily heard at the commencement of auscultation and may radiate over a wide area of the chest wall; it does not produce a thrill.
4/6	Murmur readily heard at commencement of auscultation and is accompanied by a thrill.
5/6	Very loud murmur, heard with the stethoscope barely touching the chest but becomes inaudible when the stethoscope is lifted just clear of direct contact with the chest. It is accompanied by a thrill.
6/6	Very loud murmur, it is heard even when the stethoscope is not in direct contact with the chest wall. It is accompanied by a thrill.

Murmurs included in this category are those that occur in the absence of other signs of cardiovascular disease and which may or may not be pathological, and may warrant reassessment at a later date (Table 11.4).

Thrill

A thrill is a palpable vibration which accompanies the more intense murmurs. It can be felt by placing the palm of the hand on the thoracic wall. Usually the site of thrill coincides with the point of maximum intensity of a murmur. A murmur associated with a thrill is usually pathological.

Table 11.4 Murmurs of doubtful significance

Grade 3/6 systolic murmurs on the left thoracic wall in adult racing thoroughbreds and in hunters.
Grade 3/6 systolic murmurs in horses under the influence of sedatives. Murmur may disappear when influence of sedative has worn off.

On rare occasions a thrill may occur because of arteriovenous anastomoses in peripheral tissues. As arteriovenous anastomoses can give rise to heart failure, they should be surgically corrected where feasible.

HEART RATE

The resting heart rate in the horse is usually in the range of 28–40 beats/min. It varies because it is influenced by many factors such as age, breed, body size and, in mares, the stage of gestation. In very fit, lightweight breeds (racehorses) the resting rate may be only 24 beats/min. Rates as low as 20 have been recorded from a horse in training and may indicate excessive vagal tone. Certainly in untrained, unfit horses, rates as low as these would be considered abnormal and warrant an electrocardiographic examination.

A persistently elevated resting rate of 60 or more beats/min in adult horses may be associated with congestive heart failure. In foals, the heart rate in congestive heart failure is usually in the range of 80–240 beats/min.

The heart rate recorded from normal racing thoroughbreds during maximal exercise is slightly over 240 beats/min. It takes at least 1 h after cessation of exercise for the rate to return to its pre-exercise level; in some normal horses it may be several hours. While the rate of recovery may be influenced by many variables, the recovery rate following submaximal exercise appears to be more rapid in the fit than in the unfit subject.

RHYTHM

On clinical examination up to 20% of racehorses may have irregular heart rhythm. In the smaller breeds the percentage is lower. Much of the irregularity is because of heart block and is usually ascribed to the strong influence exerted by the vagus nerve on the equine heart. Other causes are atrial fibrillation, premature beats and tachycardia.

Atrioventricular heart block

This results from defective conduction of the electrical signals from the atria to the ventricles. There are three degrees of block.

(1)   First degree, which is an abnormal prolongation of the atrioventricular conduction time. It is essentially an electrocardiographic diagnosis.
(2)   Second degree, where the signal periodically fails to reach the ventricles and the heart drops a beat.
(3)   Third degree, where there is complete failure of atrioventricular conduction. The atria beat normally, but the ventricles rely on a subsidiary pacemaker and beat much more slowly and out of step with the atria.

Third degree block is not commonly encountered in the horse. It is a pathological condition. It should be suspected in a horse with a very slow heart rate which does not significantly increase with exercise. Also, there may be a history of fainting attacks. It is advisable to carry out an electrocardiographic examination in any severe bradycardia.
First and second degree block frequently occur together. Unless severe, they are usually regarded as benign. Second degree block can be diagnosed clinically when the heart rate is slow by the presence of pauses (dropped beats) in the rhythm and the occurrence of an atrial sound (S4) near the beginning of the pauses. In most cases, the heart block disappears when the heart rate accelerates to 50–60 beats/min. It should be noted that dropped beats may also occur in normal horses as a transitory phenomenon shortly after exercise when the heart is beginning to slow down. One should be careful not to confuse the irregular rhythm caused by benign atrioventricular heart block with that associated with atrial fibrillation or vice versa.

Atrial fibrillation

Atrial fibrillation is the most common cause of gross irregularity in the rhythm of the equine heart. It is a state where the atria display continuous electrical activity but fail to pump.

Fortunately, only a limited amount of this very rapid electrical activity is relayed to the ventricles. Ventricular activation is erratic; this explains much of the irregular rhythm encountered in atrial fibrillation.

On auscultating the heart the rhythm is usually grossly irregular; short and long pauses occur at random. Some of the pauses may be preceded by a few rapidly occurring beats. The intensity of S1 may vary markedly. The heart rate is usually 30–40 beats/min but may occasionally be in excess of 200. With very rapid rates a pulse deficit may be detected, i.e. the heart rate determined from the heart sounds at the chest is greater than the rate determined concurrently from the arterial pulse. Atrial fibrillation may be transient or chronic. Two main problems present themselves with atrial fibrillation.

(1) During strenuous exercise the horse may tire easily, stumble and fall.
(2) The horse may die suddenly, either during strenuous exercise or while at pasture.

Atrial fibrillation may occur in association with underlying cardiac disease, or cardiac disease may not be present. Where the condition is not associated with underlying cardiac disease, quinidine sulphate given orally may restore normal rhythm. In some horses it may recur.

A paroxysmal form of atrial fibrillation may occur in racehorses. It persists for only a short time after racing; in the majority of horses it disappears within 24 h after the race, and may not recur.

Premature beats

Premature beats are recognized when a regular rhythm is interrupted by beats occurring sooner than anticipated; in many instances they are followed by a relatively long pause. They may occur regularly or irregularly, frequently or infrequently, and as isolated beats or in groups of two or three. In most instances premature beats occur at rest and disappear with exercise, in others they appear with or shortly after exercise or excitement.

Depending on their site of origin in the heart, there are

two types, ventricular and supraventricular. Supraventricular premature beats occur more commonly than ventricular premature beats. Both types may or may not be associated with organic heart disease. Isolated premature beats may occur in normal horses when excited. When they occur frequently, and especially if in groups, they may be associated with underlying heart disease. An electrocardiographic examination may provide more information here. Not infrequently, premature beats disappear if the horse is given a few months of rest. The significance of premature beats should be judged in the context of the overall physical health of the animal, and the presence or absence of murmurs according to the dictum "judge them by the company they keep".

Tachycardia

Tachycardia simply means a rapid heart beat. There are three types: sinus, supraventricular and ventricular.

In sinus tachycardia, beats are normal but occur at a rapid rate (above the arbitrary value of 50 beats/min). A bout of sinus tachycardia begins and ends gradually. It occurs in exercise, with fear or excitement. It may also occur as part of a compensatory mechanism in shock and with congestive heart failure.

Supraventricular tachycardia (SVT) consists of a rapid succession of four or more supraventricular premature beats. These beats arise from a site in the heart above the level of the ventricles.

Ventricular tachycardia (VT) consists of a rapid succession of four or more ventricular premature beats. An electrocardiogram is needed to differentiate SVT from VT. SVT and VT may occur in paroxysms which may last seconds, minutes, hours or days. In contrast to sinus tachycardia, the bout begins suddenly and ends just as abruptly.

Supraventricular tachycardia may be associated with atrial enlargement or myocarditis. It may also occur during the conversion of atrial fibrillation to normal rhythm.

Ventricular tachycardia is generally considered a more ominous sign than SVT; it may more readily progress to a fatal rhythm. VT may be associated with myocarditis, septicaemia, toxaemia, and quinidine intoxication. Persistent, repetitive bouts of SVT and especially VT, should be viewed with concern. Where appropriate, treatment should be instituted. In uncomplicated cases of SVT, digoxin may be used. VT responds best to quinidine sulphate given orally. If a more rapid response is demanded, quinidine gluconate or procainamide may be given slowly by the intravenous route. Both can lower blood pressure.

RELIABLE SIGNS OF CARDIAC DISEASE (TABLE 11.5)

Table 11.5 Reliable signs of cardiac disease

*Grade 4/6 or louder, systolic murmur in the absence of anaemia.
*Prolonged grade 2 or louder, diastolic murmur.
*Precordial thrill in the absence of anaemia.
*Generalized venous engorgement.
*Atrial fibrillation.
*Third degree (complete) atrioventricular heart block.
*Premature beats occurring frequently; multi-shaped in ECG.
*Ventricular tachycardia.

CHAPTER 12

Forelimb Lameness: An Approach to Diagnosis

SUSAN J. DYSON

INTRODUCTION

Forelimb lameness in the horse is a condition commonly encountered in practice. An accurate history may often suggest the cause of lameness and, apart from obvious details such as age and breed, a number of points deserve particular attention (see Table 12.1).

Table 12.1 Important points for case history.

Length of ownership
Veterinary examination at purchase
Type and amount of work
Previous occurrence of lameness
Onset and duration of present lameness, with any preliminary signs
When last shod; uneven wear of shoes
Response to treatment by the owner

WHERE TO START

As a high proportion of lameness is related to the foot this is a logical place to start the examination. Nevertheless, lameness may originate elsewhere and it is important to carry out a thorough examination of the whole limb, starting at the top of the limb and working down, finally concentrating upon the foot. Although this sounds a lengthy procedure it takes surprisingly little time and facilitates detection of less common causes of lameness. The problem may be bilateral although appearing overtly as a unilateral lameness so examination and comparison of both forelimbs is often helpful.

The duration of lameness will, to an extent, determine the thoroughness of the first examination; if the horse has been lame for only 24 h and a careful clinical examination reveals nothing obvious, a few days box rest with or without the shoe removed may resolve the lameness. If the lameness has been present for several weeks then a more detailed investigation is warranted.

CLINICAL EXAMINATION AT REST

It is valuable to examine the horse at rest and in some instances the diagnosis may be reached without seeing the horse walk or trot. The examination is most easily performed in a stable or relatively confined space but a proper examination is difficult if the horse does not stand still. The use of a chain shank over the nose gives effective restraint (Fig. 12.1). Conformation and foot shape are best assessed with the horse standing squarely on a flat surface.

STANCE AND ATTITUDE

The way in which the horse stands may be significant. A horse with laminitis will tend to stand with the hindlimbs further under the body than usual, with the forelimbs slightly outstretched and the weight rocked back on to the heels.

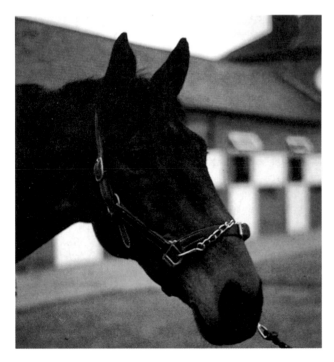

Fig. 12.1
A properly applied
chain shank provides
additional restraint.

A horse with navicular disease may stand either with straw stacked under the heels, artificially raising the heels, or with one foot slightly in front of the other (pointing) with or without the heels slightly lifted. A horse with radial nerve paralysis stands with the elbow "dropped" and in severe cases, the carpus and fetlock are semiflexed with the dorsal wall of the foot resting on the ground. This position may also be adopted by a horse with a fracture of the olecranon or after trauma to the shoulder region and these conditions must not be confused.

In the majority of lamenesses the horse's attitude is unchanged, but a horse in severe pain may be dull and show patchy sweating. Pus in the foot or infection in a joint often cause considerably more pain and distress than a fracture.

MUSCLE ATROPHY

The presence of muscle wastage can be misleading. Slight disuse atrophy of the supraspinatus and infraspinatus muscles does not ncessarily reflect shoulder lameness but may be associated with any chronic forelimb lameness.

CONFORMATION

Abnormal conformation predisposes to lameness. When viewed from the front, the "normal" forelimb is straight. Lateral positioning of the metacarpal region relative to the forearm and carpus ("bench knee") may predispose to the development of a "splint" involving the second metacarpal bone and also stresses abnormally the lower limb joints as does either toe-in or toe-out conformation. Likewise a "broken" pastern-foot axis places unnatural strain on the distal limb joints and also the suspensory apparatus.

FOOT SHAPE

Foot shape, symmetry and balance are assessed both with the foot weightbearing, when it is viewed from all angles, and non-weight bearing. The leg is picked up and held just proximal to the fetlock and the foot is allowed to hang down freely (Fig. 12.2). The foot should be trimmed so that there is a straight pastern foot axis, to which the heels of the foot are parallel. The medial and lateral halves of the foot should be symmetrical with the heels of equal height so that, when the horse is standing, the foot is on the same sagittal plane as the rest of the limb with the lower limb joints parallel to each other. If one heel is higher than the other this may predispose to bruising, damage to the sensitive laminae or disease of the lower limb joints.

Horses which have been lame for some time, either clinically or subclinically, often have asymmetrical front feet. The foot of the lame leg is narrower with more upright walls than the contralateral foot. This asymmetry may reflect both increased weightbearing by the foot of the sound limb, with spreading of the foot and decreased weightbearing by the foot of the lame limb resulting in contraction. Although this usually reflects a foot lameness, it does not do so invariably.

Although navicular disease has classically been associated with a narrow, upright, boxy foot, it is frequently seen in the

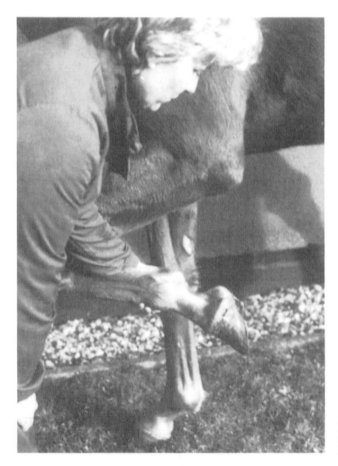

Fig. 12.2
Assessment of foot
balance.

horse with long toe and low heel conformation, with or
without collapse and contraction of the heels (Fig. 12.3). This
conformation probably predisposes to navicular disease and
osteoarthrosis of the distal interphalangeal joint and abnormally stresses the suspensory apparatus.

Assessment of foot shape and balance, and the way in
which the foot is shod, is important not only for reaching a
diagnosis but also when considering treatment. A poorly
fitted shoe can be a direct cause of lameness. If the branches
of the shoe are too short this effectively decreases the surface
area over which forces are distributed, increasing the force
per unit area. This may predispose to bruising at the heels,

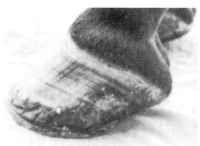

Fig. 12.3
A foot with an excessively long toe and low collapsed heel. The branches of the shoe are too short and provide no support to the heels.

especially if the heel of the shoe is poorly finished, and also gives no support to the heels which will tend to collapse. If a branch of the shoe has shifted towards the frog, or the wall is overgrowing the shoe, this can cause bruising, splitting of the hoof wall and damage of the sensitive laminae.

SWELLINGS

Each leg is viewed from all angles in order to identify any abnormal swellings. The position and extent of the swellings are related to normal anatomical structures and the limbs are compared. There are some abnormal swellings which are not necessarily clinically significant. It is not unusual for the medial palmar vein on the proximomedial aspect of the metacarpal region to be distended in sound horses (Fig. 12.4). This slight soft tissue swelling is often poorly demarcated and must not be confused with swelling around the deep digital flexor tendon or its accessory ligament (inferior check ligament).

Many normal horses have either distension of the digital flexor tendon sheaths (tendinous windgalls) and, or, distension of the fetlock joint capsules (articular windgalls). These may be unilateral or bilateral and may fluctuate in size, depending upon the amount and type of work the horse is doing, the ground conditions and the environmental temperature. Although tendinous windgalls rarely cause problems, enlargement of a fetlock joint capsule may sometimes be associated with lameness.

The site of swelling does not necessarily reflect accurately the location of the problem. There are multiple causes of

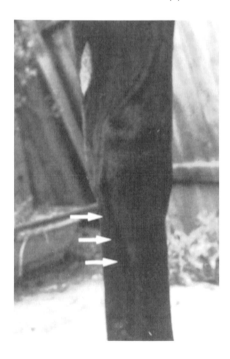

Fig. 12.4
Distension of the medial palmar vein.

diffuse soft tissue swelling in the metacarpal region (Table 12.2), including not only local pathology, e.g. cellulitis or strain of the superficial digital flexor tendon, but also problems elsewhere, e.g. oedema associated with pus in the foot. This oedema may extend proximally as far as the carpus.

PALPATION

Each leg is felt from top to bottom, both with the limb weightbearing and non-weightbearing. It is useful to establish a regular sequence for every examination, so that no structure is overlooked. The purposes are to establish the presence and nature of abnormal swellings, to detect areas of heat and to assess whether pressure applied to a site causes pain.

Many horses have firm enlargements on the second and fourth metacarpal (splint) bones and, unless pressure applied to the area causes pain, it is unlikely that the swelling is the cause of lameness.

Table 12.2 Causes of diffuse swelling in the metacarpal region.

Strain of the superficial digital flexor tendon
Strain of the deep digital flexor tendon
Sprain of the accessory (inferior check)
   ligament of the deep digital flexor tendon
Sprain of the suspensory ligament
Bruising caused by direct trauma
Cellulitis
Puncture wound
Foreign body
Fractured splint bone
Cracked heels
Pus in the foot

Interpretation of any reaction to palpation must be assessed carefully and this can be difficult in an apprehensive, hyper-reactive horse. The reaction is compared with the contralateral limb and is usually repeatable if it genuinely reflects pain.

Initial assessment of the size of the suspensory ligament and the size and contour of the flexor tendons is best done in the weightbearing limb. The width of the suspensory ligament should be uniform from top to bottom and this can be judged by running both thumbs simultaneously down the dorsal and palmar aspects of the ligament on both the medial and lateral sides of the limb. The palmar aspect of the superficial digital flexor tendon should have a straight contour. There is often a slight enlargement in the middle of the palmar aspect of the superficial digital flexor tendon, where the communicating branch between the medial and lateral palmar nerves runs and pressure applied to this nerve may cause pain.

If there is a larger discrete swelling on the palmar aspect of the superficial flexor tendon, it is important to know whether the horse has been wearing bandages or boots. Excessive pressure localized to a small area can cause peritendinous swelling and it is critical to try to differentiate this from a true tendon strain. Any enlargement of a flexor tendon should be viewed with concern, unless it is obviously firm and painless.

If a flexor tendon is damaged it is often possible to detect some alteration in its consistency and shape if the leg is held semiflexed. An acutely injured tendon is softer at the site of damage and its margins are less sharply defined than usual. Horses doing a lot of fast work, performing on hard ground or jumping, may show increased reactivity to palpation of both the suspensory ligament and the flexor tendons of each forelimb.

DIGITAL BLOOD VESSELS

The size of the digital blood vessels and the intensity of the pulse in the digital arteries are assessed by palpation at the level of the proximal sesamoid bones, with the limb weightbearing. In normal, shod, sound horses the vessels are palpable with a detectable pulse. A normal unshod horse which is turned out on hard ground, may have slightly enlarged blood vessels, with a readily palpable pulse over the digital arteries.

The vessels may be enlarged in a "footy" horse or a horse with navicular disease. There are several conditions including laminitis and infection in the foot, in which these vessels will become more prominent and have a strong, bounding pulse (Table 12.3). Comparison of the medial and lateral vessels may indicate whether a focus of infection is medial or lateral.

RINGBONE AND SIDEBONE

Firm enlargements in the pastern region must be interpreted with care. Horses may have hard, fibrous swellings which

Table 12.3 Causes of enlargement of the digital blood vessels and changes in the amplitude of the pulse.

Pus in the foot
Laminitis
Severe solar bruising
Nail prick/nail bind
Navicular syndrome
Fracture of the distal phalanx

mimic bone, but which are unassociated with lameness. Degenerative joint disease of the proximal interphalangeal joint (ringbone) can only be diagnosed definitively by radiography.

The ease with which the cartilages of the hoof can be felt above the coronary band, and their flexibility, are difficult to correlate with the degree of ossification seen radiographically. Ossification of these cartilages (sidebone) is seen in many normal horses, especially heavier hunter and cob types. The cartilages may ossify from more than one centre and separate islands of bone must not be confused with a fracture. Sidebone is rarely a primary cause of lameness, although asymmetrical ossification of the medial and lateral cartilages of the hoof may be associated with lameness related to chronic imbalance of the foot (Fig. 12.5).

JOINT CAPSULE DISTENSION

The size of the metacarpophalangeal (fetlock) joint capsules is most easily appreciated with the limb weightbearing (Fig. 12.6). Although a soft fluctuant swelling between the palmar aspect of the cannon bone and the suspensory ligament (the proximal outpouching of the fetlock joint capsule) may be present in normal horses, unilateral distention or one which is much larger in one leg than the other may be significant and reflect underlying joint disease. The absence of enlargement or

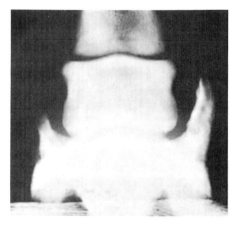

Fig. 12.5
Asymmetrical ossification of the cartilages of the foot associated with chronic foot imbalance.

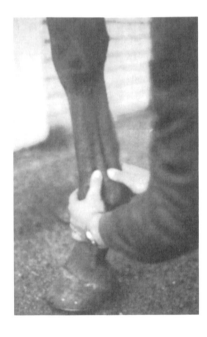

Fig. 12.6
Assessment of the width of the suspensory ligament.

distension of the joint capsule does not preclude the existence of fetlock joint disease.

Distension of the antebrachiocarpal (radiocarpal) or middle (intercarpal) joint capsules is best appreciated by viewing the carpus obliquely. Holding the leg semiflexed between one's knees, each joint space is palpated using two hands (Fig. 12.7). Subtle distension may indicate joint disease.

MANIPULATION

The range of movement and flexibility of each joint and the reaction to manipulation of the joint are assessed. Many normal horses resent pulling of the whole leg backwards or abducting the limb. The normal carpus can be flexed so that the fetlock touches the back of the elbow and resistance is significant. Resentment of slight flexion of the fetlock is highly suggestive of a fetlock problem but in some horses with fetlock pathology the joint may be flexed maximally before causing pain. The absence of a response to flexion does not exclude that joint as a potential source of pain.

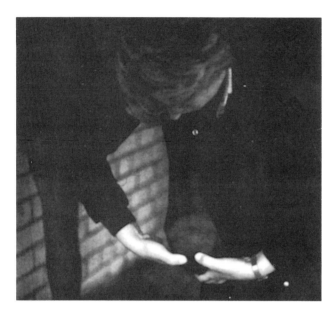

Fig. 12.7
Palpation of the
intercarpal joint
capsule.

HOOF TESTERS

Hoof testers must be used with care. It is easiest to place the
horse's leg between your own legs in order to have both
hands free to manipulate the hoof testers. In this way one
can feel if the horse reacts to applied pressure. It may be
necessary to bend your knees in towards the horse so as not
to cause discomfort by applying undue torque on the fetlock
and carpal joints.

The hoof testers are applied gently at first; a horse with
pus in the foot, or laminitis, may show considerable pain to
relatively light pressure, even thumb pressure. The area of
maximum pain is localized carefully remembering that hoof
testers apply pressure at two points. If there is infection in
the foot, it is sometimes possible to hear pus squeaking
beneath the sole as pressure is applied to it.

The consistency of the sole is assessed. The soft, readily
compressible sole is more prone to bruising than a hard,
unyielding sole, but the absence of reaction to hoof testers
does not preclude the existence of a bruise. Pressure applied
across a single heel may elicit pain caused by a corn, or a
wing fracture of the distal phalanx (pedal bone). In the

author's experience it is unusual to get a pain reaction in a horse with navicular ˙disease, unless it also has corns. Percussion applied to the wall of the foot with the limb weightbearing may identify a site of pain associated with an incorrectly placed nail, or damage to the laminae.

EXCESSIVE SWELLING

If there is considerable, diffuse, soft tissue swelling in an area, such that the individual structures cannot be palpated, and there is no obvious primary cause (e.g. pus in the foot, cracked heels or a puncture wound), it is often useful to hose the leg with cold water two or three times daily over the next 24–48 hours, to bandage the leg and to confine the horse to a box. The horse is reassessed when some of the swelling has dispersed.

An anti-inflammatory analgesic drug such as phenylbutazone (2 g twice daily for 1–2 days) is also helpful. It may then be possible to identify which structure(s) are swollen and the extent of the damage. Even at this stage it may be impossible to make an entirely accurate diagnosis or prognosis and further examination may be necessary.

EXAMINATION AT EXERCISE

Examination of the horse moving is best done on a hard, level, non-slip surface, preferably roughened concrete or tarmac. This allows the examiner both to see the way in which the horse moves and how each foot is placed to the ground, and also to listen to the rhythm. Sometimes lameness is more easily heard than seen.

The horse must be adequately restrained but the handler must interfere minimally with the horse's head movement. The horse may best be restrained in a bridle but the handler must take care not to pull excessively on the mouth via the reins.

The gait is difficult to assess if the horse is not moving forwards freely. It can be helpful to encourage the horse with a lunge whip and although the horse may at first become hurried, it usually settles quickly.

AT WALK

The horse is first observed at the walk, both from beside, behind and in front. The slow sequence of foot falls enables the examiner to watch carefully the flight of the limb, the height of the arc of the foot, and the placement of the foot to the ground, be it flat, the inside wall or outside wall first, toe first or heel first. The horse with laminitis takes short strides, tending to place the feet to the ground heels first. Repeated landing on one heel first can predispose to bruising or damage of the sensitive laminae. The horse is watched as it turns both to the left and to the right, because this may accentuate lameness, especially if it is associated with a foot problem.

AT TROT

Unless the lameness is severe, the affected limb is best identified with the horse trotting. The head nods downwards as the sound limb is weightbearing and may be lifted slightly as the lame limb bears weight but a pronounced head lift is unusual unless the lameness is very severe, or the source of pain is proximal to the carpus.

The speed of the trot is important because subtle lameness may be difficult to detect if the horse trots too fast. The stride length, foot placement and limb flight are assessed. A bilaterally short, shuffly stride is suggestive of foot pain. If the lameness is unilateral the stride length is usually not significantly shortened, unless the pain is very severe and the horse is anticipating weightbearing, or the lameness originates in the upper forelimb.

A horse with navicular disease tends to land toe first. The degree to which a fetlock sinks during weight bearing may be reduced if the joint is painful. If there is carpal joint pain, the lame limb may be swung outwards to minimize carpal flexion as the limb is advanced.

The horse should be observed for long enough to appreciate the degree of lameness and to assess whether the lameness is consistent or variable, if it improves or deteriorates with exercise. A young horse with osteo-chondrosis of the shoulder may show an extremely variable degree of lameness. Only when at its worst is the lameness characteristic of an upper forelimb lameness (shortened stride, lower limb flight, marked head lift and nod). Lameness associated with a splint may deteriorate with exercise whereas lameness caused by navicular disease is usually consistent or may improve.

FLEXION TESTS

Flexion tests are used to assess whether lameness can either be accentuated or produced. When flexing the fetlock and interphalangeal joints, the author finds it easiest to face caudally and hold the foot (Fig. 12.8). In this position it is easy to move with the horse if it moves. The joints are flexed with moderate, but not excessive pressure for approximately 30–45 s.

It is important to compare the reaction of the two limbs. The sounder of the two limbs is tested first because if the lame leg is flexed first, the lameness may be accentuated to such an extent that the reaction to flexion of the other leg is masked. If there is a significant reaction to flexion, the accentuation of lameness will be apparent despite the horse walking a couple of steps before trotting. Although the horse may need encouragement to trot freely, it should not be rushed.

A normal horse may take a few unlevel steps after prolonged flexion but more than four or five lame steps is considered significant. The test is not specific because not only will pain from the fetlock or interphalangeal joints cause an accentuation of lameness but many horses with navicular disease also show exacerbation of lameness. By holding the leg just distal to the fetlock rather than by the foot, the test becomes more specific as the fetlock joint is flexed independently of the lower joints.

Although most horses with fetlock joint problems will show increased lameness after flexion, a negative response does not preclude the fetlock joint as the source of pain. Likewise, carpal flexion may accentuate lameness associated with carpal joint pathology, but a negative response does not exclude the carpus from further investigation.

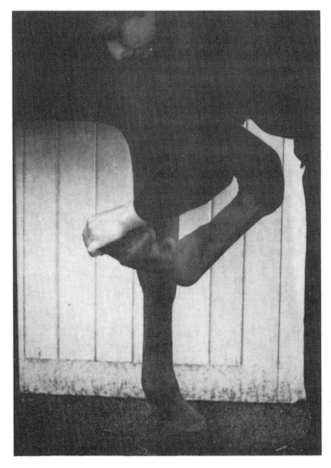

Fig. 12.8
Flexion of the fetlock
and interphalangeal
joints.

CIRCLES

Lameness which is barely detectable, or is inapparent in
straight lines, may be obvious when the horse moves in
circles, especially with the affected leg on the inside. It is
easiest to lunge the horse because many horses are reluctant
to trot in circles if led. Ideally it is useful to compare the
horse lunged both on a soft surface (grass) and a hard surface
(roughened concrete). The "footy" horse or horse with bruising
may improve substantially on a soft surface.

Lameness associated with navicular disease is usually
accentuated on a circle. The horse is lamer on the left forelimb

on the left rein and on the right forelimb on the right rein. If the horse is lamer with the affected limb on the outside of the circle, it is unlikely that the cause is navicular disease. However, other foot problems, high suspensory desmitis and shoulder lameness should be included in the differential diagnosis.

RIDDEN EXERCISE

Ridden exercise is occasionally useful but an inexperienced rider may complicate the picture by inadvertently moving his or her hands in rhythm with the trot, thus influencing the movement of the horse's head. Nevertheless, sometimes ridden exercise is invaluable for accentuating a lameness which is otherwise barely detectable.

The veterinarian must beware of drawing too many conclusions about a chronically lame horse which has been without shoes for some time. The horse may be slightly foot sore which may influence its way of moving. A horse which is in regular work may show a very different degree of lameness to a horse which has been rested for some time, and the reaction to flexion tests is likely to be greater. If the horse has been rested, and demonstrates only subtle lameness, it is often best if the horse resumes work with a view to accentuating the lameness before further investigation is carried out.

FURTHER INVESTIGATION: WHAT TO DO NEXT

At this stage, or earlier in the examination, many potential problems have been excluded, and there may be strong indications of where the source of pain is. If there is evidence of pain in the foot, it may be useful to remove the shoe and explore further. This is inadvisable if it is intended to use local anaesthesia because with one shoe on and one off, the lameness is more difficult to assess and the horse may become foot sore. If the source of lameness is unknown it is helpful to establish whether the problem originates in the foot or elsewhere and this is readily achieved by performing palmar (abaxial sesamoid) nerve blocks. If a fracture is suspected the area should be examined radiographically.

REMOVAL OF THE SHOE

Removal of a shoe without damaging the foot is easily accomplished by the veterinary surgeon, but it is acknowledged that a skilled farrier may be better able to explore the foot than an inexperienced veterinarian. If the horse has been recently shod and the clenches are well knocked down, the shoe may be removed more easily by rasping the clenches than by elevating them with a buffer. If it is suspected that lameness is related to recent shoeing, each nail is removed individually. The horse may show resentment as a nail which was placed too close to the sensitive laminae is removed.

After removal of the shoe the sole is pared and inspected for the presence of haemorrhage along the white line, separation at the white line (which may reflect higher laminar damage) and subsolar haemorrhage. The absence of visible reddening of the sole does not preclude the presence of deeper bruising and corns may be missed without paring away several of the superficial layers of horn at the heels. The hoof testers are used again to try to identify a focus of pain.

The shoe which has been removed is inspected for signs of abnormal wear. A horse with navicular disease which lands toe first may have excessive wear of this part of the shoe. The levelness of the bearing surface is assessed; an unlevel surface concentrates pressure at points, rather than distributing it evenly and this may predispose to low grade bruising.

If lameness has been present for 4 weeks or more, and has failed to respond to rest, further investigation is indicated, either by the original veterinarian or a specialist. This investigation includes local anaesthesia, radiography and, or, ultrasonography, and in many instances can be performed usefully earlier in the course of lameness. The earlier the cause of lameness is established, the more likely it is that appropriate therapy will be effective.

LOCAL ANAESTHESIA

Even after a thorough clinical examination it is frequently impossible to define accurately the source of pain without the use of regional anaesthesia, intra-articular anaesthesia or local infiltration of anaesthetic. It is a vital part of clinical diagnosis in the majority of cases of chronic lameness (more than four weeks duration) and its use may be indicated at the initial examination. Only when pain has been definitively localized to an area either by clinical signs and, or, by local anaesthesia can radiographs be interpreted properly.

This subject is considered in detail in Chapter 14 and will only be discussed briefly. The horse must be lame enough to block, so that improvement can be assessed, and each block must be tested to ensure that it has worked before its effect on lameness is judged. It is important to be sufficiently selective as opposed to being satisfied with making the horse sound.

Although a horse with navicular disease is rendered sound by desensitizing the entire foot by palmar (abaxial sesamoid) nerve blocks, many other causes of lameness are also improved by these blocks. A horse with navicular disease is usually sound after desensitizing of only the palmar (caudal) part of the foot by bilateral palmar digital nerve blocks. It must also be remembered that this block is not specific for navicular disease but can relieve pain associated with other conditions such as soft tissue damage.

Just occasionally the results of local anaesthesia are misleading, and if the clinical examination suggests strongly that, for example, pain originates in the foot, radiography of this area is indicated even if the horse was not rendered sound by apparent desensitization of the region. If there is extreme pain it may be impossible to eliminate lameness by regional anaesthesia (e.g. some cases of pus in the foot).

RADIOGRAPHIC EXAMINATION: WHERE AND WHEN TO X-RAY

In most circumstances, radiographs are only useful once pain has been definitively localized to an area. Many normal horses show radiographic changes which are not clinically significant and which can only be interpreted in the light of the results of a detailed clinical examination. Small osteophytes may be present on the dorsoproximal aspect of the proximal phalanx which do not always indicate clinically significant fetlock joint disease.

There may be many small radiolucent areas along the distal

border of the navicular bone, which represent nutrient foramina and synovial outpouchings and do not necessarily indicate navicular disease (Fig. 12.9). Thus radiographs are used to support or refute the clinical diagnosis. It must be remembered that the absence of significant radiographic abnormalities involving a joint does not preclude that joint as the site of pain. There are horses in which pain can be localized to the fetlock joint by regional and intra-articular anaesthesia, which show no radiographic changes.

If the clinical signs are suggestive of a fracture then the suspected area should be radiographed before local anaesthesia is employed. If a horse has laminitis and has been lame for some time before examination, or is failing to respond to treatment, then lateral radiographic views of each foot are useful to assess whether or not the distal phalanges have rotated and how much horn can be safely removed by trimming in an attempt to restore a more normal orientation of the bones.

To be of any value there must be a sufficient number of radiographic views of diagnostic quality (see Table 12.4). Two views of a joint are not enough to determine that there is no significant pathology. The area to be X-rayed is suitably prepared to avoid the presence of confusing artefacts. Mud is brushed off and if a foot is to be examined the shoe is removed to avoid obscuring the margins of the distal phalanx. After trimming and scrubbing the foot it is useful to pack the frog clefts with a slightly radio-opaque substance, such as

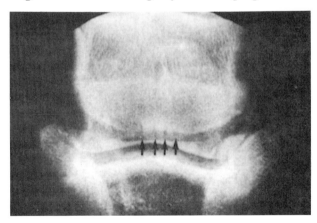

Fig. 12.9
Dorsopalmar radiographic view of the navicular bone of a sound horse. There are several radiolucent areas along the distal border of the navicular bone.

Table 12.4 Essential views for radiographic examination of the distal forelimb.

Area	View	*kV	mAs	Notes
	Lateromedial	75	4.0	Lysholm focused grid (8:1)
Foot	Dorsopalmar (upright pedal)			
	(1) Distal phalanx	65	2.0	Lucidex focused grid (6:1)
	(2) Navicular bone	75	4.0	Lysholm 8:1 focused grid. Frog packed with
	(× 2)			Play-Doh
	Palmaroproximal-palmarodistal oblique	70	3.2	
	Lateromedial	65	4.0	
Pastern/fetlock	Dorsopalmar	65	5.0	
	Dorsopalmar lateromedial	65	3.2	
	Dorsopalmar mediolateral	65	3.2	
	Dorsopalmar	65	5.0	
Second and fourth	Dorsopalmar lateromedial oblique	60	2.5	
metacarpal bones	Dorsopalmar mediolateral oblique	60	2.5	
	Flexed lateromedial	65	4.0	
Carpus	Dorsopalmar lateromedial oblique	65	4.0	
	Dorsopalmar mediolateral oblique	65	4.0	

*These exposure factors are approximate. All views obtained using high definition screens and appropriate film.

Play-Doh, to eliminate confusing frog cleft shadows.

Coning down the primary beam reduces scatter and this both improves definition and reduces the radiation hazard. Although grids can also be useful to improve definition of a picture, especially in a dense area such as the navicular bone region, it must be remembered that the use of a grid requires higher kV and mAs and a longer exposure time increases the risk of movement blur.

Each cassette is labelled using X-ray sensitive paper on which is written the name of both the horse and the owner, and the date of examination. Appropriate lead markers are attached so that each view can be clearly identified. Dark room technique is critical and errors may spoil otherwise adequate films. Nevertheless, with attention to these details it should be possible to obtain good quality views of the carpus and distal limb with a small portable machine, but if this is impractical the horse should be referred elsewhere.

The radiographs are viewed both on a viewing box and over a bright light otherwise subtle abnormalities may be missed. Active periosteal proliferative reactions and newly developed osteophytes are not very radio-opaque and tend to be overexposed, but can be identified over high density illumination. It is often useful to compare similar views of the normal, contralateral limb. For example, separate centres of ossification of the dorsoproximal aspect of the proximal phalanx may be present bilaterally unassociated with lameness and should not be confused with chip fractures. The interpretation of radiographs requires a good knowledge of radiographic anatomy and its variations and if there is any doubt then the films should be referred for a second opinion.

ULTRASONOGRAPHY

Ultrasonography is invaluable for objective appraisal of soft tissue swellings of the distal limbs or for further investigation of an area to which pain has been localized. As with radiographs high quality images are essential for accurate diagnosis. The limb must be prepared appropriately by fine clipping or shaving, washing and liberal application of a coupling gel. High detail images of relatively superficial structures are needed, therefore a 7.5 MHz transducer (linear or sector scanner) is required. Appropriate gain controls must be used so that the outline and internal architecture of each structure is readily appreciated. In order to examine the most superficial structures (e.g. the superficial digital flexor tendon) it is essential to use a stand off. Both transverse and longitudinal images of the area in question should be obtained, and carefully labelled, permanent records should be made using either a thermal printer or a Polaroid camera. It is impossible to interpret poor quality images. Just as with radiographs, it is important to have a good knowledge of anatomy; if there is any doubt concerning interpretation it is generally preferable for the horse to be referred for a second opinion.

DIAGNOSIS

A logical and systematic approach to lameness investigation usually results in an accurate diagnosis or at least in localizing pain to an area. If it is not possible to be more specific about the cause of lameness, there is little to be gained by allocating the condition a name. With the available techniques, it is sometimes impossible to be more accurate. Nevertheless, every effort must be made to be as specific as possible. For example, pain in the foot is often attributed to pedal osteitis, which is probably an over-diagnosed condition. There is tremendous variation in the normal radiographic appearance of the distal phalanges and many normal horses have irregular borders of the bone, broad vascular canals and a large crena at the toe. The term pedal osteitis should be restricted to those horses with periosteal proliferative reactions on the dorsal surface of the bone, seen in a lateral view, and, or, multiple circular radiolucent areas within the bone, seen in the dorsopalmar (upright pedal) view. If pain is localized to the foot and there is no obvious diagnosis based on the clinical examination and radiography, the next logical step is to anaesthetize the distal interphalangeal joint for which specialist help may be required.

In many instances, sophisticated diagnostic techniques are unnecessary and lameness diagnosis is well within the scope of the thoughtful, thorough, non-specialist investigator. If unable to reach a satisfactory conclusion either because of a lack of equipment or experience, specialist advice should be sought because the longer the duration of lameness, the poorer the long term prognosis tends to be.

CHAPTER 13

Forelimb Lameness: Diagnosis and Treatment

SUSAN J. DYSON

INTRODUCTION

In Chapter 12 methods of approach for the investigation of forelimb lameness were discussed. In this chapter a number of common causes of lameness are considered in more detail and methods of treatment are outlined. Although some of these treatments are beyond the scope of the general practitioner, it is important to be aware of what can be done and to decide when specialist help is required.

PUS IN THE FOOT

Pus in the foot (underrun sole) is the most common cause of lameness.

DIAGNOSIS

A presumptive diagnosis may be made from the clinical signs (Table 13.1). In some cases it may not be possible to locate pus, although pain can usually be localized to a discrete area. Occasionally a nerve block is useful to confirm that pain originates from the foot. It is often not possible to identify a route of entry of infection, however, hoof wall cracks are a common site. Black areas in the white line should be regarded with suspicion as a possible focus of infection.

TREATMENT

Remove the shoe and pare the sole over the area of maximum pain until pus is released or until a black area in the white line is cut out completely. If the sole is extremely hard, it may help to poultice the foot for 48 h (hot Animalintex; Robinsons) to soften the sole. Athough a large enough hole must be created to allow drainage, exposure of an excessive amount of sensitive tissue will delay the horse's return to work. It may be best to create a moderately sized hole and poultice the foot for several days. Infection is usually caused by anaerobic bacteria and it is useful to flush the hole with an oxidizing agent such as hydrogen peroxide.

Table 13.1 Pus in the foot: clinical signs.

History	Lameness may be sudden or gradual in onset
Clinical examination	Moderate to very severe lameness; horse may be reluctant to move and may be sweating and blowing. In the early stages lameness may be intermittent and slight.
	"Bounding" digital pulses (compare medial and lateral).
	May be diffuse oedematous swelling of the distal limb up to and including the metacarpal region.
	Foot usually warmer than the contralateral foot.
	May be slight softening at a localized area of the coronary band (site where pus likely to break out).
	Hoof testers cause pain over a variably sized area (unless the sole is excessively hard).
	Pus may be heard squeaking beneath the sole when pressure is applied to the sole; the sole may be unusually soft over a localized area.

In very severe cases local treatment with metronidazole (Torgyl; RMB) is extremely useful and obviates the need to pare the foot excessively. Approximately 5 ml is injected into the hole daily for 3 or 4 days. Sometimes no pus is released when the foot is pared but after poulticing for several days the lameness resolves. Systemic antibiotics are rarely required and may delay recovery, but tetanus prophylaxis is mandatory using tetanus toxoid or, if the vaccination status is unknown, tetanus antitoxin.

While the moist, sensitive tissues of the sole are exposed they must be protected and kept clean and dry. Chlortetracycline (Aureomycin; Cyanamid) spray is useful to harden these areas after resolution of infection. If the horse is to be turned out, a shoe may provide some protection if the lesion is close to the wall. A large solar defect may be protected temporarily by either a thick metal plate or a leather pad. It is preferable to cover only the affected area and not the whole sole.

Long standing infection in the foot can result in infectious osteitis of the distal phalanx, which can be diagnosed radiographically as a radiolucent area in the margin of the bone seen in a dorsal palmar (upright pedal) view. Surgical treatment is usually necessary.

GENERAL TRAUMA WITH SECONDARY INFECTION (TABLE 13.2)

TREATMENT

Clip the hair around the wound and thoroughly clean it with a suitable antiseptic such as dilute iodine solution (Previdine Scrub; Berk). If the wound is severely contaminated, preliminary hosing may be helpful. Debride the wound if necessary. If the wound is of puncture type, a hot poultice may help to "draw" the infection. Depending on the nature and extent of the wound, a dry, nonadherent dressing (Melolin; Smith & Nephew) gamgee and a crepe bandage can be applied provided that the area is accessible to bandaging. Change the dressing daily.

Systemic antibiotics (procaine penicillin G, 22 000 iu/kg

Table 13.2 General trauma with secondary infection: clinical signs.

History	The horse is generally found in a field with a "big leg" or has been treated unsuccessfully and, or, inappropriately for a known wound.
Clinical examination	Diffuse, warm swelling.
	Oedema
	Cellulitis
	Pain on pressure over localized or more diffuse area.
	Wound(s) (may be necessary to clip hair to identify nature and extent of wounds).
	Pus may be present.
	Moderate to severe lameness.
	May be depressed, inappetent and pyrexic.

NB. If the wound is in the proximity of a joint or tendon sheath it is critical to establish whether either have been penetrated. Infection within a synovial structure may have devastating consequences without appropriate treatment. If this is suspected, the horse should be referred immediately to a specialist for lavage of the synovial structure and aggressive antimicrobial therapy

intramuscularly once a day with, or without, neomycin 5 mg/kg intramuscularly) should be administered daily for 5 days. If possible, confine the horse to a box or covered yard. It is important that tetanus prophylaxis be carried out.

COMPLICATIONS

If infection is not resolved completely within 5 days, or if no improvement is observed after 3 days of treatment, swabs should be collected from the wound for aerobic and anaerobic bacterial culture and appropriate antibiotic sensitivity testing.

While awaiting the bacterial culture results, antimicrobial therapy may be changed to intravenous oxytetracycline 5 mg/kg once a day. If the wound is a deep, puncture type, or is discharging foul smelling pus, suspicious of infection by anaerobic bacteria, it may be flushed daily with approximately 5–8 ml metronidazole for 3 or 4 days.

If appropriate antimicrobial therapy still fails to resolve the infection, radiography should be performed to identify bony changes typical of infectious osteitis, osteomyelitis or sequestrum formation and to preclude the presence of a radio-opaque foreign body. Surgical exploration is indicated if neither are identified.

CORNS

Corns are a common cause of slight lameness, especially on hard ground. Poor trimming and shoeing or inadequate frequency of shoeing predispose a horse to corns (Fig. 13.1). The condition must be differentiated carefully from lameness due either to early navicular syndrome or to bad shoeing per se (Table 13.3).

DIAGNOSIS

If the horse is sound after palmar digital nerve blocks and if there is a single corn at either the medial or the lateral heel, desensitization of that heel should render the horse sound. After removal of the shoe and paring of the sole, redness (subsolar haemorrhage) can be seen at the "seat of the corn" (Fig. 13.2).

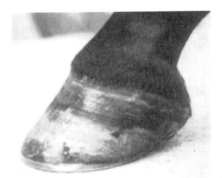

Fig. 13.1
The foot is overgrowing the shoe and this may predispose to corns. This shoe was originally shaped to fit the curve of the wall exactly. If the shoe had been fitted slightly wide at the heels it would have accommodated some foot growth. The branch of the shoe is rather short and the heel of the shoe concentrates pressure on the "seat of corn".

Table 13.3 Corns: clinical signs.

History	Gradual or sudden onset of mild to moderate lameness; worse on hard ground, especially on turns.
	Often occurs several weeks after shoeing.
	May be unilateral or bilateral.
Clinical examination	Shoe may obviously fit badly, or be overgrown by the foot.
	May be a slight increase in intensity of the digital pulses.
	May be pain caused by pressure with hoof testers at the heel(s)
	Short stride; lamer when turning.
	Obvious lameness on circle with lame leg on inside, especially on hard ground.

TREATMENT

Remove the shoe for 24–48 h and poultice the foot. Advise that the foot be trimmed correctly and reshod appropriately. The branches of the shoe should be sufficiently long and correctly finished. If the branches are too short, they may

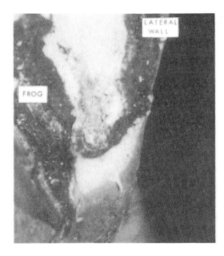

Fig. 13.2
Reddening of the sole at the "seat of corn" reflecting previous subsolar haemorrhage (bruising). It may be necessary to pare off several layers of horn before subsolar haemorrhage becomes visible.

concentrate pressure at the seat of corn.

The horse may benéfit from a wide webbed shoe with a concaved solar surface (a "seated out" shoe) which protects the seat of corn without placing pressure on it directly (Fig. 13.3). Advise that the horse must be shod regularly at intervals of no more than 6 weeks and possibly more frequently if the foot grows rapidly. It is usually unnecessary to shoe the horse with pads. Pads themselves may create problems and their use is to be avoided if possible. With a pad it is more difficult to fit a shoe correctly and the foot tends to sweat abnormally, the horn quality deteriorates and grit may accumulate beneath the pad.

NAIL BIND OR PRICK (TABLE 13.4)

DIAGNOSIS

Remove the shoe by removing each nail individually. The horse may resent removal of the offending nail. Lameness is often much improved after removal of the shoe.

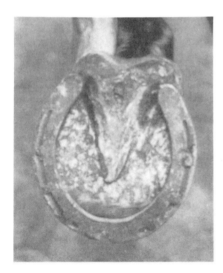

Fig. 13.3
A broad webbed flat shoe with a concaved solar surface (a seated out shoe). The shoe provides some protection to the sole without applying pressure to it.

Table 13.4 Nail bind or prick: clinical signs.

History	Recently shod (within 5 days).
	Slight to moderate lameness, especially when turning.
Clinical examination	May be increased density of digital pulse medially and, or, laterally.
	Pain caused by pressure or percussion with hoof testers, especially percussion over the head of the offending nail.

TREATMENT

Flush the hole with hydrogen peroxide or iodine solution (50%). Poultice the foot for 24 h and then replace the shoe.

THE NAVICULAR SYNDROME (TABLE 13.5)

The incidence of navicular syndrome is much higher in horses than in ponies. It occurs in all sizes and shapes of feet but a small foot relative to body size may predispose to the syndrome. In Great Britain it is seen most often in horses with long toe and low heel conformation.

DIAGNOSIS

The horse may be sound after medial and lateral palmar digital nerve blocks, but contralateral limb lameness may then become apparent. This may not be obvious when the horse moves in straight lines, but is revealed when the horse moves in circles. Radiography is used to support the clinical diagnosis; significant abnormalities include large radiolucent areas in the middle of the navicular bone, multiple triangular shaped, flask shaped or irregularly shaped radiolucent areas along the distal straight and sloping borders of the navicular bone, new bone on the proximal border of the navicular bone and an abnormal contour of the navicular bone seen in a true lateral view (Fig. 13.4). The palmaroproximal-palmarodistal oblique view may

Table 13.5 The navicular syndrome: clinical signs.

History	Decreased stride length and unwillingness to go forward freely.
	Stiffness, especially when first coming out of box.
	A jumping horse may stop uncharacteristically.
	Intermittent, slight shifting forelimb lameness or more obvious unilateral lameness.
	Lameness usually insidious in onset and may initially improve during an exercise period.
	Lameness usually improves with prolonged rest but recurs when regular work is resumed.
	Lameness or shortening of stride, worse on hard ground especially when turning.
Clinical examination	May "point" the foot at rest.
	Enlarged digital blood vessels.
	Usually no reaction to hoof testers unless corns also present.
	Lameness may be very slight to moderate, unilateral or bilateral.
	Tendency to land toe first.
	Lameness accentuated as horse turns.
	Lameness may be worse after fetlock flexion.
	Lameness more obvious on inside forelimb on lunge.

show narrowing of the flexor cortex, new bone formation on the flexor surface, loss of trabecular pattern within the medullary cavity with sclerosis and poor corticomedullary definition.

It is helpful to radiograph both feet; the radiographic abnormalities may be more obvious in the less lame foot. Some horses with slight clinical signs have minimal radiographic abnormalities; some sound horses have multiple radiolucent areas along the distal border of the navicular bone. Occasionally discrete osseous or mineralized bodies on the distal border of the navicular bone are seen in sound horses. Radiography is only helpful if combined with a careful clinical examination.

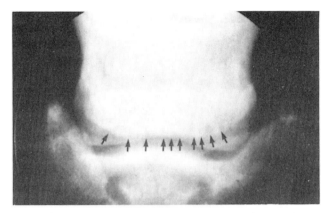

Fig. 13.4 Dorsopalmar (upright pedal) radiographic view of the navicular bone of a horse with navicular disease. There are multiple variously shaped and sized radiolucent areas along the distal straight and sloping borders of the navicular bone (arrows).

TREATMENT

Appropriate trimming and shoeing

Balance the foot and shorten the toes. Set the shoe wide and long at the heels and set the toe of the shoe back and, or, roll the toe of the shoe (Fig. 13.5). An egg bar shoe can be useful especially for a very badly shaped foot. Benefits of this shoe include increased support for the heels and an increased weightbearing surface (Fig. 13.6). Avoid the use of wedge pads to raise the heels artificially; although temporarily beneficial, pads tend to discourage development of a better shaped heel. The aim is to achieve a normal foot conformation. If the foot is poorly balanced and misshapen it may take 12–18 months of careful foot care before the ideal is approached. Collaboration with a skilled, cooperative farrier is essential. Combine treatment with regular work and, if necessary, drugs or surgery.

Drugs

Phenylbutazone

This drug is palliative only, but a combination of appropriate shoeing, analgesic medication and regular work may break

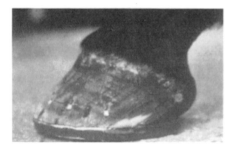

Fig. 13.5
A well dressed and shod foot. The toe is short and the dorsal wall of the foot and the heel are approximately parallel. The shoe is slightly set back at the toe and the branches of the shoe are set wide and extend beyond the ground surface of the heels. There are no nails caudal to the quarters of the foot, so expansion of the heels is not restricted.

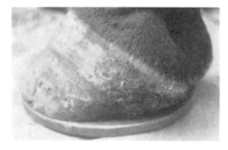

Fig. 13.6
An egg bar shoe with a rolled toe. The shoe provides additional support for severely collapsed heels.

the vicious cycle of poor blood flow in the foot, lameness, irregular work, poor blood flow. Try 1 g twice daily by mouth. If the horse is not substantially improved within 3–6 months (i.e. moves more freely without medication), alternative treatments should be considered as delay may reduce the long term prognosis.

Isoxsuprine (a peripheral vasodilator)

Give 0·6 to 0·9 mg/kg twice daily by mouth for a minimum of 6 weeks followed by a reducing dosage regimen (0·3 to 0·4 mg/kg twice daily for 3 weeks; 0·3 to 0·4 mg/kg twice daily on alternate days for 3 weeks). The drug is helpful in approximately 50% of horses, but about half of these relapse within 2–3 months of completing a course of treatment. A second course may be helpful (the higher dose rate is recommended). The long term response after withdrawal of treatment is variable (fair to poor).

Warfarin (reduces plasma viscosity; an anticoagulant)

Start with a dose rate of 0·02 mg/kg once daily by mouth. Because of its anticoagulant properties, warfarin is a potentially hazardous drug and the one stage prothrombin time (a measure of clotting function) must be monitored regularly (twice weekly during the stabilization period and then monthly). The one stage prothrombin time must be measured before treatment is started. Thereafter the aim is to increase by approximately 25% the pretreatment one stage prothrombin time; if this is not achieved and the horse is still lame, the dose of warfarin should be increased by approximately 10% until there is satisfactory prolongation of the one stage prothrombin time. Improvement in lameness is seldom observed in less than 6–8 weeks.

Some horses respond clinically to treatment although the prothrombin time is not significantly prolonged compared to pretreatment. According to Colles (1979), this drug is effective in up to 75% of horses but continual treatment is required for 12–18 months. Subsequently about 50% of cases can cease treatment successfully. The author's experience has been much less favourable.

Surgery

Palmar digital neurectomy

The horse will only at best be as sound as it is after palmar digital nerve blocks. This is a relatively simple surgical procedure but potential complications include failure of desensitization caused by an aberrant nerve supply, formation of painful neuromas, regeneration of nerves and reinnervation of the foot and degenerative changes in the deep digital flexor tendon. Good hygiene and foot care are mandatory postoperatively to avoid potentially disastrous complications such as unrecognized infection in the foot. Approximately 75% of horses will remain sound for up to 18 months.

Desmotomy of the collateral (suspensory) ligaments of the navicular bone

The surgical procedure should be carried out in the distal pastern region to avoid complications associated with the proximal interphalangeal joint. The success rate is at most 75% in the short term, declining with time. It is not possible to predict pre-operatively which horses may respond to treatment.

COMMENTS

In some horses with appropriate trimming, shoeing and work, with or without medication, lameness associated with navicular syndrome is manageable, at least in the short term. Progress cannot reliably be monitored radiographically; no improvement of the lesions is seen in successfully treated horses.

CRACKED HEELS (TABLE 13.6)

TREATMENT

Clip the hair and clean the area thoroughly, removing scabs. Apply a soothing cream with antibiotics and corticosteroids

Table 13.6 Cracked heels: clinical signs.

History	Occurs in stable kept and pastured horses, especially during winter. Large amount of feather may predispose to the condition.
Clinical examination	May be diffuse oedematous swelling of the metacarpal region.
	Swelling on the palmar aspect of the pastern with crusted, excoriated cracks in the skin (may be difficult to see without trimming the feather).
	Resentment of flexion.
	Stiff gait: may be moderately lame.

topically (e.g. Dermobion; Willows Francis Veterinary, or a mixture of Cetavlex; ICI: sulphanilamide powder and prednisolone). Occasionally systemic antibiotic therapy is useful. The affected area must be kept clean and dry. Provide tetanus prophylaxis.

LAMINITIS (TABLE 13.7)

Laminitis occurs most commonly in small overweight ponies. It also occurs in horses, when the prognosis is much more guarded. Front feet are most commonly affected but hind feet may be involved either alone or with front feet.

DIAGNOSIS

Clinical signs are diagnostic, except in mild cases. If lameness is severe or refractory to treatment or if there is a history of

Table 13.7 Laminitis: clinical signs.

History	Onset usually, but not always, associated with the consumption of rich grass (especially in spring and autumn), or overconsumption of grain.
Clinical examination	Horse is reluctant to move and stands with the hind feet further under the body than usual, with the forelegs slightly outstretched and the weight rocked back on to the heels. Mild cases may show only slight stiffness.
	Prominent digital pulses (may involve hind feet as well as front feet). Feet warm (or cold).
	Pain on pressure with hoof testers in toe region and on percussion of the wall.
	May be very prominent rings on wall of foot which diverge at the heels reflecting previous episodes of laminitis (may influence prognosis).
	Feet may be misshapen; high heels, long toe, concave dorsal face of wall (also indicative of previous attacks).
	Horse moves with shuffly gait placing the feet to the ground heel first.

previous laminitis, lateral radiographic views of the feet are useful to determine if there is rotation of the distal phalanges and to assess how much foot can be trimmed safely. (This is also beneficial for public relations between veterinary surgeon and farrier.)

TREATMENT

Starvation

Either confine the horse to a very small paddock with minimal grass and no supplementary feeding, or confine to a box with non-edible bedding (e.g. woodshavings) and feed a maximum of 1·5 kg hay twice daily (one small wedge twice daily).

Anti-inflammatory analgesics

Give phenylbutazone by mouth – start the treatment intravenously (Table 13.8). The risk of side effects of phenylbutazone therapy (oral and gastrointestinal ulceration, diarrhoea) is much greater in ponies than in horses.

The drug may be administered either in a very small quantity of oats, bran or barley or mixed with water or milk of magnesia and administered by syringe. Flunixin meglumine (Finadyne; Schering-Plough) is an equally effective drug, but is considerably more expensive.

Table 13.8 Suggested dosage regimen for phenylbutazone

450 kg bodyweight horse	Day 1	2 g twice daily
	Day 2	2 g and 1 g
	Days 3–7	1 g twice daily
200 kg bodyweight pony	Day 1	2 g
	Day 2	1 g twice daily
	Days 3–7	0·5 g twice daily

Additional dietary supplements

This is helpful in some horses, especially recurrent cases: methionine (5–10 g daily), potassium chloride (15 g per day), sodium chloride (15 g per day) and calcium carbonate (30 g per day).

Acepromazine

In the acute stage horses and ponies have associated hypertension; acepromazine (0·04 mg/kg) reduces blood pressure and may have beneficial clinical effects.

Foot trimming

Shorten the toe as much as possible and lower the heels. Radiographs are a useful guide (Fig. 13.7). An overlong toe acts as a lever and tends to cause more separation of the laminae. In the acute stage the horse is usually best left either with, or without, shoes as it was before the onset of lameness.

Daily walking exercise

Walk the horse for 10 min several times a day.

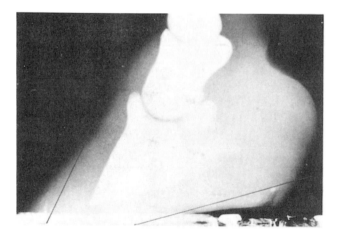

Fig. 13.7 Lateral radiographic view of a foot of a pony with laminitis. The toe of the distal phalanx has rotated distally. The toe of the foot is excessively long and the heels are too high. The lines indicate approximately how much of the foot can be removed safely.

Local analgesia

If the pain is uncontrollable by systemically administered drugs, palmar (abaxial sesamoid) nerve blocks can be helpful three times per day. Bupivacaine, being relatively long acting, is the local anaesthetic of choice. (Theoretically, decreased pain results in decreased catecholamine release and reduced vasoconstriction). This may increase the risk of rotation of the distal phalanx and if the pain is so severe it may indicate that further investigation and treatment of a primary systemic problem is required.

FRACTURE OF THE DISTAL PHALANX (TABLE 13.9)

DIAGNOSIS

Lameness is alleviated by palmar (abaxial sesamoid) nerve blocks. A unilateral block may be sufficient. In a dorsopalmar (upright pedal) radiographic view a radiolucent line orientated differently to the vascular channels is usually seen. The shoe must be removed and the foot cleaned before radiography. In the acute stage there is minimal separation along the fracture line so the fracture may be difficult to identify. Oblique radiographic views may be helpful (Fig. 13.8).

Table 13.9 Fracture of the distal phalanx: clinical signs.

History	Usually sudden onset of moderate to severe lameness either during exercise or when turned out in a field.
Clinical examination	May be increased intensity of digital pulses.
	Resting pain.
	Usually pain caused by pressure with hoof testers over region of fracture.
	A moderate to severe lameness accentuated by turning.

If a fracture is not seen but the clinical signs are typical, the horse should be treated as if it has a fracture and the foot re-radiographed after 7–10 days. Rarefaction along the fracture line occurs as a normal part of the healing process so a fracture may be seen more easily at this stage. It is important to assess whether or not there is displacement of the fracture, if it is articular or nonarticular, and how much of the joint surface is involved.

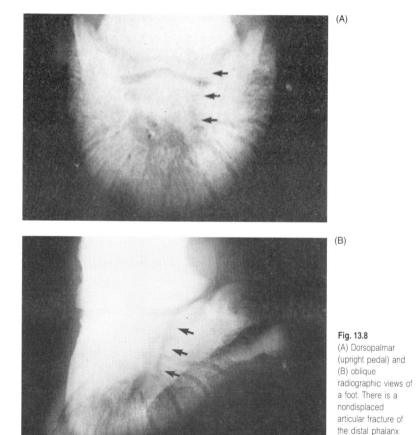

(A)

(B)

Fig. 13.8
(A) Dorsopalmar (upright pedal) and (B) oblique radiographic views of a foot. There is a nondisplaced articular fracture of the distal phalanx (arrows).

TREATMENT

Box rest the horse for a miminum of 3 months. Shoe the foot with a bar shoe (Fig. 13.9) with a cross bar across the affected heel and, or, additional side clips close to the fracture site. This immobilizes the distal phalanx as much as possible. Analgesics should be administered as necessary to minimize the risks of the development of laminitis in the contralateral foot secondary to excessive weight bearing. The foot should be radiographed again after three months but the fracture may heal by fibrous union and may still be detectable. It is useful to continue to shoe the horse with a bar shoe when it is returned to work. Selected intra-articular fractures may benefit from internal fixation but this is technically difficult and there is a high incidence of postoperative sepsis.

SECONDARY (DEGENERATIVE) JOINT DISEASE OF THE PROXIMAL INTERPHALANGEAL JOINT: RINGBONE (TABLE 13.10)

DIAGNOSIS

Lameness is improved considerably by palmar (abaxial sesamoid) nerve blocks but the horse is rarely sound. The

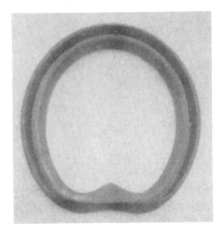

Fig. 13.9
A bar shoe, appropriate for a horse with a "wing" fracture of the distal phalanx. The bar shoe immobilizes the hoof wall as far as is possible.

Table 13.10 Secondary joint disease of the proximal interphalangeal joint: clinical signs.

History	Unilateral or bilateral lameness of variable duration and severity; lameness may be intermittent and deteriorate with work.
Clinical examination	There may or may not be palpable firm swelling in the pastern region at the level of the proximal interphalangeal joint (firm, fibrous swellings can mimic bony enlargements and may be present without lameness). Radiography is essential to make a diagnosis.
	May be resentment of passive flexion or of twisting the joint.
	Variable degree of lameness which is usually worse on hard ground and may be accentuated on a circle.
	Lameness exacerbated after flexion.

horse is usually sound after palmar (mid cannon) and palmar metacarpal nerve blocks. Radiography is essential – dorsopalmar, lateromedial and oblique views (Fig. 13.10). Significant abnormalities include periosteal proliferative reactions, narrowing of the joint space, subchondral bone sclerosis and subchondral radiolucent areas. There is often roughening on the dorsal aspect of the middle phalanx of no significance (Fig. 13.11). There may be additional periosteal proliferative reactions which are non-articular and of lesser significance. The absence of radiographic changes does not preclude early secondary joint disease.

TREATMENT

Treatment depends on the severity of radiographic abnormalities and is generally palliative only.

(1) If radiographic changes are minimal and the lameness is improved by intra-articular anaesthesia of the joint, intra-articular medication with sodium hyaluronate or a glycosaminoglycan (Adequan; Luitbold-Werk) could be considered.
(2) If obvious radiographic abnormalities are present phenyl-

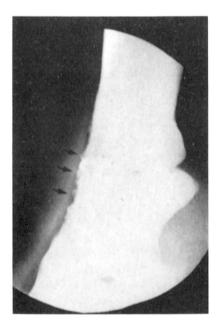

Fig. 13.10
Lateral oblique radiographic view of the proximal interphalangeal joint of a horse with secondary joint disease (ringbone). There are slight periosteal reactions on the articular margins of the proximal and middle phalanges (arrows).

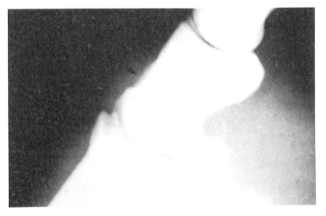

Fig. 13.11 Lateral radiographic view of the proximal interphalangeal joint of a normal horse. There is some roughening of the contour of the dorsal aspect of the middle of the middle (second) phalanx (arrow) of no clinical significance.

butazone may be administered to effect to alleviate pain. Some benefit may be achieved by the intra-articular administration of a corticosteroid, although this may accelerate degradative changes and treatment may have to be repeated.

(3)   Surgical arthrodesis could be considered but the outcome is less favourable than in a hindlimb.

SPRAIN OF THE FETLOCK JOINT

DIAGNOSIS

The diagnosis is based upon the clinical signs (Table 13.11). Radiographic examination is useful to identify chip fractures and should certainly be performed if the horse fails to respond to treatment within 7 days or if lameness recurs when work is resumed.

TREATMENT

Local hot and cold treatment for 2–3 days is helpful to reduce soft tissue swelling (cold hosing and hot poultices). Local ultrasound treatment is also effective. Bandage the leg to try to maintain the reduction in soft tissue swelling and confine the horse to a box until all the soft tissue swelling has resolved. Anti-inflammatory analgesics may be beneficial. Hand walking exercise may start when the acute inflammation has resolved. The horse should improve considerably within a few days and after a mild sprain can often resume work after 10–14 days. Intra-articular administration of sodium hyaluronate

Table 13.11 Sprain of the fetlock joint: clinical signs.

History	Sudden onset of lameness.
Clinical examination	Distension of fetlock joint capsule with or without periarticular soft tissue swelling.
	Local heat.
	Pain caused by flexion of joint.
	Moderate degree of lameness.

(Hylartil; Pharmacia) may accelerate recovery, especially in a horse which has failed to improve with conservative treatment.

PERIOSTITIS OF THE SECOND AND FOURTH METACARPAL BONES ("SPLINTS") (TABLE 13.12)

DIAGNOSIS

The clinical diagnosis may be confirmed by infiltration of local anaesthetic around the site of the "splint". Radiography is usually unnecessary unless a swelling is very large and a fracture is suspected, but can be useful for differentiating between an active "splint" (roughened periosteal reaction, see Fig. 13.12) and an inactive "splint" (smoothly outlined bony enlargement) and for monitoring progress.

Table 13.12 Periostitis of the second and fourth metacarpal bones: clinical signs.

History	Gradual or sudden onset of slight to moderate lameness which deteriorates with work, especially on hard ground.
	All ages of horses affected, but most common in young horses (3–6 years old).
Clinical examination	May be obvious or only subtle enlargement over splint bone (second metacarpal bone more commonly affected than fourth).
	Swelling usually comprises some bone reaction and some overlying soft tissue reaction. Subtle swellings may only be identified by careful palpation with the limb non-weightbearing.
	Pressure applied to localized area of the bone causes pain (the reaction is compared with the contralateral limb).
	Moderate degree of lameness which may be accentuated by prolonged pressure over the "splint".

TREATMENT

Box rest (approximately 6 weeks) with, or without, local injection of corticosteroids. In some horses lameness associated with a "splint" takes an unusually long time to resolve.

STRAIN OF THE SUPERFICIAL OR DEEP DIGITAL FLEXOR TENDON (TABLE 13.13)

TREATMENT

The aim of treatment is to reduce soft tissue swelling as quickly as possible and this can be achieved by ice and cold water therapy and systemic administration of phenylbutazone for 24–48'h, keeping the leg bandaged between treatments. Local ultrasound or laser treatment can be helpful. Confine the horse to box rest. A course of a glycosaminoglycan

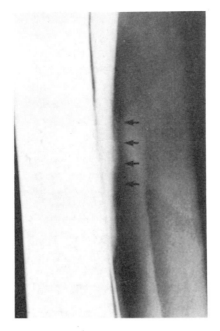

Fig. 13.12
Lateral oblique radiographic view of the metacarpal region projecting the second metacarpal bone. There is an active periosteal proliferative reaction ("splint") (arrows).

Table 13.13 Strain of the superficial or deep digital flexor tendon: clinical signs.

History	Sudden onset of swelling (localized or diffuse) with, or without, lameness. A discrete small swelling of the superficial flexor tendon may be present without lameness. This is often an "early warning sign" and if the horse is kept in work a more severe and obvious strain is likely to occur.
Clinical examination	Superficial digital flexor strain: Abnormal contour of the superficial flexor tendon (best assessed with the leg bearing weight).
	Deep digital flexor: Swelling of the deep digital flexor tendon. (Strain of the deep digital flexor tendon is very rare and swelling in this region usually reflects sprain of its accessory ligament, the inferior check ligament.) If there is too much swelling, it is impossible to make an accurate diagnosis. The limb is treated by cold hosing and applying a firm bandage. An anti-inflammatory drug, e.g. phenylbutazone, is administered and the limb is re-examined within 24–28 h
	Palpation of the tendon reveals a localized or diffuse enlargement of the tendon with rounding of its contour. It feels softer than usual. Digital pressure applied to the primary site of damage usually causes pain (compare contralateral limb).
	Slight to severe lameness depending on the degree of damage.
	Diagnostic ultrasonography is useful to identify the extent of injury especially in mild cases.

polysulphate (Adequan; Panpharma) administered intramuscularly may be beneficial. When the acute inflammation has subsided cold water therapy can cease and short periods of hand walking exercise can start after 7–10 days. At this stage, try removing the bandage for a few hours but if swelling recurs, it should be replaced. Keep the horse in with daily walking exercise for a minimum of 6 weeks before being turned out for further convalescence. Alternatively the horse may be placed in a small yard or paddock where it will do no more than walk. The total rest period required is approximately 12 months.

If a swelling of the superficial flexor tendon is very localized it may be the result of direct trauma or an overtight bandage. The damage may be only peritendinous and the convalescence time can be shorter. Diagnostic ultrasound is the best method of differentiation between a peritendinous and a tendinous lesion.

CHAPTER 14

Nerve Blocks and Lameness Diagnosis

SUSAN J. DYSON

INTRODUCTION

Although the importance of a thorough and objective clinical examination cannot be overemphasized, the use of local anaesthesia is an integral part of lameness investigation to confirm the site or sites of pain.

The results of the clinical examination may be misleading; fetlock flexion may exacerbate markedly the degree of lameness but this is a non-specific test because the proximal and distal interphalangeal joints are, inevitably, stressed concurrently.

Selective local anaesthesia helps in choosing which area to X-ray or examine ultrasonographically, and in the interpretation of radiographic abnormalities which may or may not be clinically significant.

PREREQUISITES FOR DIAGNOSIS

There are two prerequisites: an accurate knowledge of relevant anatomy and a lame horse.

The anatomy is most readily appreciated by performing a dissection and comparing the position of the nerves relative to palpable landmarks. Although the majority of horses have a uniform pattern of innervation of the limb, variations occur and this must be remembered when considering the limitations of regional anaesthesia.

The horse must be lame enough to assess the effect of local anaesthesia on the gait. Interpretation of the nerve block can be extremely difficult if the lameness is subtle. The horse should be worked for a sufficient length of time to ensure that the lameness does not improve spontaneously. The ideal surface on which to evaluate lameness is usually a flat, hard surface, so that both sight and hearing can be used to assess the lameness.

The horse may be more lame if observed moving in a circle, especially if the lameness is bilateral; the majority of horses move more freely on the lunge than if led in a circle. In some cases the lameness may be more obvious if the horse is ridden.

A skilled rider may be able to help assess the effect of the nerve block, but a less talented rider may inadvertently interfere with the horse thus making interpretation more difficult. In a horse which is only slightly lame, but shows a markedly positive response to flexion of a joint or joints, analgesia of a selected joint is sometimes useful, but it is occasionally misleading. The response to flexion may be abolished, whereas the original, mild lameness persists unchanged.

SELECTION OF LOCAL ANAESTHETIC

The selection of local anaesthetic and the amount used depends on the site to be blocked. The aim is to be as specific as possible, therefore a minimal quantity of local anaesthetic should be employed. This should also help to reduce any adverse reactions to injection.

The use of anaesthetic with or without adrenalin is debatable. Theoretically, the addition of adrenalin aids specificity since the drug is localized at the site of injection, but it also prolongs the local accumulation of the anaesthetic, making an adverse reaction more likely.

Lignocaine is the most commonly used local anaesthetic, but in some horses it is associated with marked local reactions, especially in the metacarpal region and is not the ideal drug.

In the author's opinion the best commercially available drug currently available in Great Britain is mepivacaine (Carbocaine; Fisons, or Intra Epicaine; Arnolds). An alternative is prilocaine (Citanest; Astral). Both these drugs have a rapid onset of action and are associated with minimal local reactions.

EQUIPMENT AND TECHNIQUE

The method of administration and the position of the limb depend largely on personal preference and the site to be blocked.

Either a dental syringe or needle and syringe may be used. If the latter is used, an eccentrically placed nozzle is helpful; the syringe should have a smooth nozzle rather than a Luer-Lok fitting. Needle size depends on the site to be blocked. A needleless pressure injector as used in blood transfusion units is considered by some a very valuable instrument, particularly when dealing with fractious horses. It introduces a small intradermal bleb of local anaesthetic through which a needle can be inserted very precisely, thus reducing the risk of stimulating a sudden movement by touching the nerve, or of penetrating an adjacent vessel. The author usually uses a needle and syringe.

Other materials required are scissors and, or, clippers and equipment to clean the site thoroughly. It is debatable whether it is necessary to clip the hair, but identification of landmarks is essential and this may be facilitated by removal of excessive hair.

Nerve blocks are ideally performed in a clean environment with the horse standing on a non-slip floor. Although the horse may be more easily restrained if confined in a loosebox rather than outside, the bedding should be swept to one side to avoid the frustration of searching for a needle inadvertently dropped.

Many horses tolerate the placement of needles surprisingly well but the technique is often performed more easily if the horse is restrained by a twitch.

Occasionally mild sedation is necessary. In such circumstances a small dose of xylazine should be used as its sedative effect wears off rapidly so that it will not unduly influence the horse's subsequent gait.

The needle should be inserted through the skin swiftly. The syringe is then attached. It is not necessary to aspirate before injection because if the needle is in a blood vessel, blood will rapidly appear in the needle hub. If this occurs, the needle should be withdrawn slightly.

The depth to which the needle is inserted depends on the anatomical position of the nerve. Whenever a needle is redirected, it should be withdrawn before redirection to avoid bending and weakening the needle.

Nerve blocks should be performed in a logical sequence, starting in the most distal part of the limb and working proximally. The following descriptions outline a suitable sequence. There will be instances when it is most sensible to start, e.g. by desensitizing the whole foot, rather than just the palmar aspect – this will depend on the results of the clincal examination.

If a fracture is suspected, it is usually contraindicated to desensitize the area, because of the risk of the fracture becoming displaced, comminuted or compound.

If the horse is unshod and is foot sore, there may be confusion in interpretation of the block and the situation should be avoided whenever possible. The horse should be adequately protected against tetanus.

TESTING THE BLOCK

The block is usually effective within about 5 min, but deep sensation may not be completely eliminated and up to 20 min may be necessary before the block can be properly assessed. Nerve blocking is time consuming, if performed diligently.

Loss of skin sensation is not always synonymous with loss of deep sensation and vice versa. Therefore it may be difficult to assess whether or not the block has taken effect. Every attempt should be made, especially in the distal limb, to be sure that the block has worked.

A blunt instrument, e.g. a ball point pen, is best for testing loss of sensation. It may be useful to cover the horse's eye and to approach the animal from the opposite side, so that it does not anticipate being prodded.

Some horses show remarkable lack of sensitivity, even before being blocked; this should be assessed before performing the block or a comparison made with the opposite leg.

Some areas seem uniformly more sensitive, e.g. between the bulbs of the heels. If the horse has shown pain during compression of the foot with hoof testers, the loss of this reaction is a useful way to asses the efficacy of a foot block.

An effective block may encourage the horse to drag a toe, particularly in the hindlimb. Sometimes an effective block appears to exacerbate the lameness.

SELECTIVITY

While the block is taking effect the horse may be walked to accustom it to use a partially desensitized limb, but the author does not consider this essential and usually allows the horse to stand still to discourage diffusion of local anaesthetic from the site of injection. Despite apparent cutaneous desensitization lameness may not be alleviated as soon as the horse is observed moving. The horse should be trotted several times and preferably lunged before the nerve block is deemed negative. It is preferable to reassess the horse moving in the circumstances under which it previously appeared most lame. Lameness is not always alleviated totally; improvement is generally significant. An incomplete response may be due to inability to alleviate all the pain from a single source, a mechanical contribution to lameness, or more than one source of pain.

INTRA-ARTICULAR ANAESTHESIA

Regional anaesthesia permits localization of pain to an area, as does local deposition of anaesthetic around a suspected lesion. Intra-articular anaesthesia is an important complementary technique.

Indications for intra-articular anaesthesia include:

(1) To enable a more specific diagnosis after the localization of pain to an area by regional anaesthesia.
(2) Joint effusion.
(3) Pain on passive motion of the joint.
(4) Limited range of motion of the joint.
(5) Exacerbation of lameness by flexion of a joint.
(6) In the upper forelimb (e.g. elbow and shoulder joints) where regional anaesthesia is impractical.

RADIOGRAPHY

Having localized pain to an area, a radiographic and, or, ultrasonographic examination should be performed to try to define the nature of the problem.

The owner should be forewarned that local inflammatory reactions sometimes develop secondarily to the deposition of local anaesthetic. Bandaging the leg for at least 12 h after blocking (and longer if necessary) often helps to minimize such a reaction. If a severe reaction develops, poulticing the area and the administration of phenylbutazone may aid resolution of the inflammation. In the author's experience, such reactions are rare.

NOMENCLATURE

Some confusion has arisen over the nomenclature of nerves and nerve blocks and in this chapter Nomina Anatomica Veterinaria terminology is adopted.

Sites for desensitization

The distribution of nerves in the distal forelimb are illustrated. The approximate site for desensitization of (1) the caudal one third of the foot, (2) the whole foot and part of the pastern, (3) the fetlock and distal structures and (4) the metacarpal region are indicated in Figs. 14.1 and 14.2.

DESENSITIZATION OF THE PALMAR THIRD OF THE FOOT – PALMAR DIGITAL NERVE BLOCK

(1) This is easily performed with the limb non-weightbearing (Fig. 14.3).
(2) The caudal digital nerves lie just dorsal to the superficial digital flexor tendon, closely associated with a palmar digital vein and artery and the ligament of the ergot.
(3) The lower the block is performed, the more specific it is likely to be.
(4) Using a 16×0.5 mm (25 gauge, $\frac{5}{8}$ in) needle, 1–2 ml of local anaesthetic is deposited subcutaneously. (Excessive resistance to injection probably indicates the needle is intra-dermal and should be inserted a little deeper.)
(5) Skin sensation around the bulbs of the heels is usually removed; if the block is performed more proximally, skin sensation may be lost more cranially.

INDICATIONS

Conditions affecting the palmar third of the foot which may be improved by desensitization include shoeing problems, bruising, abscess, thrush, navicular disease complex, fracture of the navicular bone, fracture of the distal phalanx, laminar tears, desmitis of the navicular ligaments, distal interphalangeal joint pain and deep digital flexor tendonitis.
   Distal interphalangeal joint pain sometimes requires desensitization of the whole foot to render the horse completely sound. The position of a fracture of the distal phalanx will influence whether or not a horse is improved by desensitization of the palmar part of the foot.

DESENSITIZATION OF THE FOOT AND PASTERN – PALMAR (ABAXIAL SESAMOID) NERVE BLOCK

(1) This is most easily performed with the limb non-weight-bearing (Fig. 14.4).

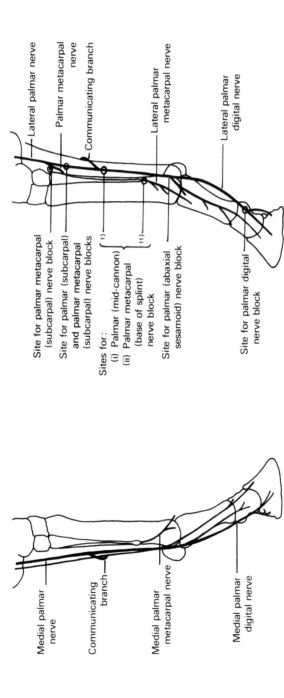

Lateral palmar nerve

Palmar metacarpal nerve

Communicating branch

Lateral palmar metacarpal nerve

Lateral palmar digital nerve

Site for palmar metacarpal (subcarpal) nerve block

Site for palmar (subcarpal) and palmar metacarpal (subcarpal) nerve blocks

Sites for:
(i) Palmar (mid-cannon)
(ii) Palmar metacarpal (base of splint) nerve block

Site for palmar (abaxial sesamoid) nerve block

Site for palmar digital nerve block

(b)

Medial palmar nerve

Communicating branch

Medial palmar metacarpal nerve

Medial palmar digital nerve

(a)

Fig. 14.1 (a) Medial and (b) lateral aspects of left distal forelimb.

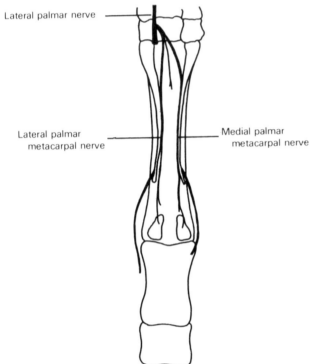

Lateral palmar nerve

Lateral palmar
metacarpal nerve

Medial palmar
metacarpal nerve

Fig. 14.2
Palmar aspect of the
metacarpal region.

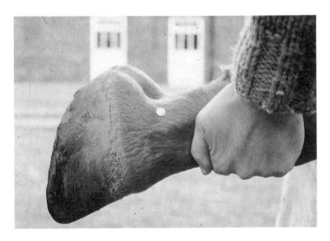

Fig. 14.3
Site for a palmar
digital nerve block.

(2)   The palmar nerve lies caudal to the vein and artery and is readily palpable over 'the abaxial surface of the proximal sesamoid bones.
(3)   Using a 16 × 0.5 mm (25 gauge, $\frac{5}{8}$ in) needle, 1–2 ml of local anaesthetic is deposited subcutaneously.
(4)   Skin sensation around the whole coronary band is usually removed.

INDICATIONS

Conditions affecting the foot and pastern which may be improved by desensitization of the region include (also see above) shoeing problems, bruising, infection, seedy toe, laminitis, fracture of the distal phalanx, keratoma, distal or proximal interphalangeal joint pain, subchondral bone cyst, laminar tears, distal sesamoidean ligament strain and some others.

Lameness associated with infection may not be totally relieved by desensitization of the foot. Proximal interphalangeal joint pain may be alleviated but may require a more proximal block to render the horse completely sound. This block may be useful in the treatment of a horse with laminitis.

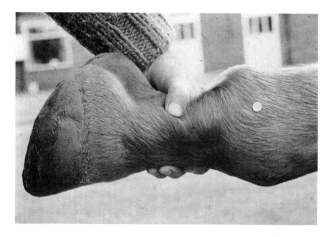

Fig. 14.4
Site for a palmar
(abaxial sesamoid)
nerve block.

DESENSITIZATION OF THE FETLOCK AND PASTERN – PALMAR (MID CANNON) AND PALMAR METACARPAL NERVE BLOCK

(1)   This is most easily performed with the limb weightbearing (Fig. 14.5).

(2)   The medial and lateral palmar nerves lie superficially between the suspensory ligament and the deep digital flexor tendon; a communicating branch is readily palpable on the caudal aspect of the limb. The palmar metacarpal nerves provide some innervation to the fetlock joint and are most easily blocked just distal to the "button" of the splint bones.

(3a)   Palmar nerves – using a 16 × 0.5 mm (25 gauge, ⅝ in) needle, 1–2 ml of local anaesthetic is deposited subcutaneously in the mid cannon region medially and laterally (NB, more proximally the nerves lie beneath the superficial fascia).

(3b)   Palmar metacarpal nerves – using a 38 × 0.6 mm (23 gauge, 1½ in) needle, 1 ml of local anaesthetic is deposited at the depth of, and just distal to, the button of each splint bone.

(4)   Skin sensation over the fetlock and pastern is usually lost; resentment to passive flexion of the fetlock is eliminated.

INDICATIONS

Conditions affecting the pastern or fetlock which may be improved by desensitization of the region include proximal

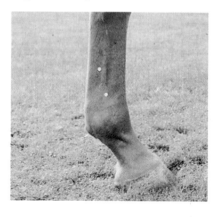

Fig. 14.5
Sites for palmar (mid cannon) and palmar metacarpal (base of splint) nerve blocks.

interphalangeal joint pain, osseous cyst-like lesions (proximal phalanx, MC3), metacarpophalangeal joint pain, collateral ligament strain, sesamoiditis, fractures of the proximal sesamoids, proximal phalanx or third metacarpal (cannon) bone and others.

Horses with a fracture may be improved significantly, although not rendered completely sound.

DESENSITIZATION OF THE METACARPAL REGION – PALMAR AND PALMAR METACARPAL (SUB-CARPAL) NERVE BLOCK

(1)   In some horses, the palmar metacarpal nerve which gives rise to both medial and lateral palmar metacarpal nerves (Fig. 14.6), and is derived from the ulnar nerve, is palpable distal to the ligament running between the accessory carpal bone and the proximal metacarpus on the lateral aspect of the carpus. The nerve lies beneath the superficial fascia. Infiltration of 2–3 ml of local anaesthetic over this nerve desensitizes the deep structures of the metacarpal region (i.e. the suspensory ligament, the accessory ligament of the deep digital flexor tendon (inferior check ligament) and second and fourth metacarpal (splint) bones and their interosseous ligaments).

(2)   If this nerve is not palpable, the deep structures can be desensitized by infiltration of about 6 ml of local anaesthetic deeply, medial to the head of the fourth metacarpal bone. With the leg non-weightbearing, a bleb of local anaesthetic is placed subcutaneously, just palmar to the head of the lateral splint bone.

A 38 × 0.8 mm (21 gauge, 1½ in) needle is directed medially to the head of the lateral splint bone and dorsally; after aspiration to check that the needle is not in a synovial structure, approximately 3 ml of local anaesthetic is injected; if there is excessive resistance to injection the needle should be withdrawn slightly. After detaching the syringe, the needle is withdrawn and redirected more medially and another 3 ml of local anaesthetic injected. The efficacy of these blocks cannot be reliably tested.

(3)   To desensitize the entire metacarpal region, it is necessary to infiltrate local anaesthetic over the medial and lateral palmar

nerves; 2 ml per site should be adequate. The nerves lie beneath the superficial fascia at this level (Fig. 14.1).
(4)   Cutaneous desensitization of the distal limb is not reliably achieved.
.(5)   The palmar aspect of the middle carpal joint capsule extends distally into the metacarpal region; subcarpal nerve blocks may alleviate lameness associated with the middle carpal joint and this joint should be blocked separately.

INDICATIONS

Conditions affecting the metacarpal region which may be improved by desensitization of the area include tendonitis or tenosynovitis, suspensory ligament desmitis, inferior check ligament desmitis, "splints", fracture of the second or fourth metacarpal (splint) bones, sore shins, stress fracture of the third metacarpal bone and others.

DESENSITIZATION OF THE CARPUS AND DISTAL LIMB – ULNAR AND MEDIAN NERVE BLOCKS

---

(1)   The ulnar nerve gives rise to the lateral palmar nerve and the palmar metacarpal nerve; sometimes desensitization of

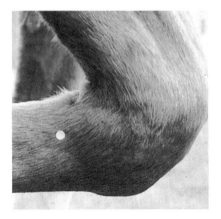

Fig. 14.6
Site for a palmar and palmar metacarpal (subcarpal) nerve block.

the latter fails to effectively eliminate lameness because of a problem in the metacarpal region, whereas an ulnar nerve block may do so.

(2)   The ulnar nerve lies beneath the superficial fascia, caudal to the deep fascia in a readily palpable groove between the ulnaris lateralis and flexor carpi ulnaris muscles, on the caudal aspect of the limb, and is most easily blocked about 10 cm (one hand's breadth) proximal to the accessory carpal bone (Fig. 14.7), with the horse weightbearing. Using a 25×0.8 mm (21 gauge, 1 in) needle, approximately 10 ml of local anaesthetic is deposited just beneath the superifical fascia.

(3)   The only area of the skin in the distal limb receiving innervation from the ulnar nerve alone is the craniolateral aspect of the metacarpus (Fig. 14.8).

(4)   The median nerve may be blocked in one of two locations:

   (a) The median nerve can be located on the medial aspect of the forearm, caudal to the radius and deep to the superficial pectoral muscle. The nerve is superficial to the brachial artery (Fig. 14.9).

   With the horse weight-bearing, after palpation of the caudal border of the radius and the distal border of the superficial pectoral muscle, a 38×0.8 mm (21 gauge, $1\frac{1}{2}$ in) needle is inserted upwards and inwards ($20°$ to the vertical) at their intersection and approximately 10 ml of local anaesthetic is infiltrated. If blood appears in the hub of the needle, the needle is withdrawn slightly before injecting.

   (b) Further distally in the forearm the median nerve lies deep to the flexor carpi radialis muscle. After palpation of the caudal border of this muscle on the medial aspect of the leg, approximately 10 cm proximal to the chestnut, a needle is inserted and directed obliquely cranially towards the back of the radius. The nerve lies behind the artery and veins; if blood appears in the hub of the needle, the needle is withdrawn slightly before injecting approximately 10 ml of local anaesthetic.

(5)   The only area of skin in the distal limb receiving innervation from the median nerve alone is the craniomedial aspect of the pastern.

INDICATIONS

The author usually finds it useful to first block the ulnar nerve and assess the effect, and if negative, then block the median nerve.

Conditions affecting the carpus which may be improved by median and ulnar nerve blocks include carpal joint arthrosis, intercarpal ligament strain, fracture, subchondral bone cyst, carpal tunnel syndrome and others.

The musculocutaneous nerve supplies cutaneous innervation only to the distal limb, therefore it is not necessary to block this nerve. Both median and ulnar nerve blocks are best

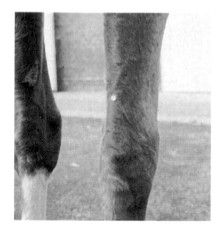

Fig. 14.7
Site for an ulnar nerve block.

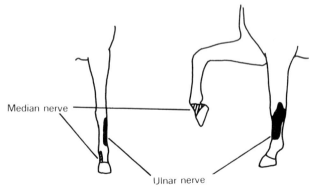

Fig. 14.8
Clinically testable areas of cutaneous desensitization for median and ulnar nerve blocks.

Median nerve

Ulnar nerve

Table 14.1 Intra-articular analgesia of the distal limb joints of the forelimb.

Joint	Site of injection	Position of limb	Volume of local anaesthetic (ml)	Needle size	Notes on technique	Time after which block best evaluated (min)	Comments
Distal inter-phalangeal	Dorsal midline approx. 2–3 cm proximal to coronary band	Weightbearing	6	0.8 mm (21 G) 38 mm	Advance the needle slowly, directing it slightly backwards. Synovial fluid usually appears spontaneously. If the contralateral limb is picked up to provide additional restraint it should be put down before the needle is removed, since it results in raised pressure within the injected joint.	5	Delayed response may reflect diffusion in the region of the navicular bone
Metacarpo-phalangeal	Palmar pouch	Semi-flexed	6–8	0.8 mm (21 G) 38 mm	Synovial fluid is much more readily retrieved if the limb is held semi-flexed. It may be necessary to aspirate. Inserting the needle through the collateral lateral ligament may reduce the incidence of iatrogenic haemorrhage.	10–30	

Joint	Site	Position	Depth	Needle	Notes	Volume (ml)	Communication
Middle carpal	(1) Dorsal aspect between tendons of extensor carpi radialis and common digital extensor	Semi-flexed	6–8	0.8 mm (21 G) 38 mm	Often necessary to aspirate synovial fluid. Think carefully about the orientation of the bones to avoid iatrogenic cartilage damage	10–30	Communicates with the carpometacarpal joint
	(2) Palmar aspect on palmarolateral aspect of limb, distolateral to accessory carpal bone	Weightbearing	6–8	0.8 mm (21 G) 38 mm	Usually necessary to aspirate synovial fluid.	10–30	
Antebra-chiocarpal	Dorsal aspect between tendons of extensor carpi radialis and common digital extensor	Semi-flexed	6–8	0.8 mm (21 G) 38 mm	Often necessary to aspirate synovial fluid. Think carefully about the orientation of the bones to avoid iatrogenic cartilage damage	10–30	No communication with middle carpal joint

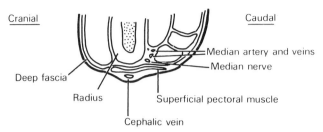

Fig. 14.9 Horizontal cross section of the medial aspect of the proximal forearm demonstrating the position of the median nerve.

performed on a different occasion from lower limb nerve blocks in order to be able to test loss of cutaneous sensation in the distal limb.

If there is clinical evidence of a carpal joint problem, it is preferable to perform more specific intra-articular anaesthesia of the suspected joint.

INTRA-ARTICULAR ANALGESIA

It is beyond the scope of this article to discuss the methods for intra-articular analgesia of each forelimb joint, therefore comment is restricted to the principles employed and a description of the methods used by the author for entering the carpal joints, the metacarpophalangeal and distal interphalangeal joints (Table 14.1). Although there is a significant risk of introducing infection into a joint when performing intra-articular analgesia, if appropriate precautions are taken the risk is considered to be very small. These precautions include:

(1) clipping a small area of hair;
(2) thoroughly scrubbing the area;
(3) appropriate restraint of the horse;
(4) use of sterile technique;
(5) use of a fresh bottle of local anaesthetic.

Equipment required includes a large gauge needle for aspiration of local anaesthetic from the bottle, sterile needles for injection (at least two), suitably sized sterile syringes and a fresh bottle of local anaesthetic, and sterile surgeon's gloves.

If working with inexperienced persons it is easiest to fill the syringe alone. The surgical glove packet is opened and laid out as a sterile field onto which two syringes are dropped. One glove is put on and a syringe picked up. Using the other hand and teeth, a large gauge (1.2 mm minimum) needle is opened and placed on a syringe. The local anaesthetic is drawn up. The needle is left in the bottle. Two suitably sized needles are opened and likewise placed on the two syringes and the needle caps removed. The syringes and needles are placed on the sterile field while the other glove is put on. The sterile field can be lifted up and placed on the ground near the horse.

INJECTING THE LOCAL ANAESTHETIC

The horse is restrained using a twitch and, if appropriate and necessary, the contralateral limb is picked up. The site for injection is carefully palpated and firm pressure applied before advancing the needle through the skin and into the joint. In some cases synovial fluid will appear spontaneously in the needle hub but it may be necessary to attach the empty syringe and aspirate, to confirm that the needle is within the joint. If the joint is markedly distended the author aspirates several millilitres of synovial fluid prior to injection of local anaesthetic, but if the joint is not distended, only a small volume of synovial fluid is withdrawn to confirm the needle's location. If synovial fluid is not readily obtained the needle is partially withdrawn and redirected. The author does not inject antibiotics but does instruct the owner of the horse that immediate advice should be sought if the lameness deteriorates within the following 48 h.

EVALUATING THE BLOCK

The speed of response to intra-articular analgesia in the forelimb is variable ranging from 5–30 min (see Table 14.1). If the block is effective a significant improvement in the lameness should be appreciable although the horse may not be free from lameness. The response to flexion of the joint should also be reduced. If intra-articular pathology is severe then the degree of improvement in the lameness may be slight.

CHAPTER 15

Problems Associated with the Interpretation of the Results of Regional and Intra-Articular Anaesthesia

SUSAN J. DYSON

INTRODUCTION

The difficulties associated with the interpretation of the results of regional and intra-articular anaesthesia are discussed with reference to eight lame horses. The clinical and radiographic features of each horse are described, together with the results of anaesthesia. One horse had clinical and radiographic signs consistent with navicular disease but it was not possible to relieve the lameness. Two horses had fractures of bones within the foot but lameness was not improved by palmar (abaxial sesamoid) nerve blocks. One horse had more than one cause of lameness. Four horses had joint pathology but none responded to intra-articular anaesthesia.

ANAESTHESIA IN LAMENESS DIAGNOSIS

Although an assessment of the history and a clinical examination of a lame horse frequently reveals the cause of lameness, it is often necessary to use local anaesthesia to identify the source. There have been many descriptions of the methods of regional and intra-articular anaesthesia (Wheat and Jones, 1981; Colbern, 1984; Dyson, 1984). Theoretically it is assumed that if pain originates from an area which has apparently been desensitized by regional (perineural) anaesthesia, then a substantial improvement in the lameness should be observed. There should also be a positive response to intra-articular anaesthesia if pain originates within a joint. In the majority of horses, this does apply and thus these techniques are an important and sometimes vital part of a lameness investigation. There are some instances when these methods yield unexpected results, or results which are difficult to interpret, some of which are discussed.

For the purposes of this chapter, it is assumed that adequate cutaneous desensitization is achieved after regional anaesthesia of an area, i.e. the horse shows no reaction to firm pressure, applied via a blunt ended instrument, to the areas in which cutaneous innervation is supplied only by the anaesthetized nerves. It is also assumed that synovial fluid is retrieved before injecting local anaesthetic into a joint, thus confirming the intra-articular location of the needle, and that the horse is observed over a sufficient time to assess the effects of local anaesthetic.

REGIONAL (PERINEURAL) ANAESTHESIA

The nomenclature employed is explained in Fig. 15.1.

FAILURE TO ALLEVIATE LAMENESS DESPITE CLINICAL AND RADIOGRAPHIC SIGNS OF NAVICULAR DISEASE

A 6-year-old thoroughbred gelding had been exhibiting intermittent left forelimb lameness of variable severity for 3 months. The horse was examined on several occasions over a period of 2 months. At times it was observed to point the left front foot. It exhibited a short striding gait with slight left forelimb lameness predominant, although occasional lame steps on the right forelimb were seen. Lameness was similar in degree on

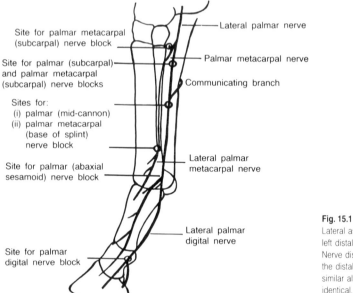

Site for palmar metacarpal
(subcarpal) nerve block

Site for palmar (subcarpal)
and palmar metacarpal
(subcarpal) nerve blocks

Sites for:
(i) palmar (mid-cannon)
(ii) palmar metacarpal
(base of splint)
nerve block

Site for palmar (abaxial
sesamoid) nerve block

Site for palmar
digital nerve block

Lateral palmar nerve

Palmar metacarpal nerve

Communicating branch

Lateral palmar
metacarpal nerve

Lateral palmar
digital nerve

Fig. 15.1
Lateral aspect of the
left distal forelimb.
Nerve distribution in
the distal hindlimb is
similar although not
identical.

hard and soft surfaces, but was accentuated when the horse
was circled towards the lame leg. Flexion of the metacarpophalangeal and interphalangeal joints slightly exacerbated the
lameness.

No method of regional anaesthesia of either the left or right
forelimb influenced the lameness. Intra-articular anaesthesia
of each of the left distal interphalangeal (coffin), humeroradial
(elbow) and scapulohumeral (shoulder) joints did not improve
the lameness.

A thorough radiographic examination of the entire left
forelimb revealed no significant abnormality, except for 10
variously shaped and sized radiolucent areas (synovial fossae)
along the distal horizontal and sloping borders of the navicular
bone, equivalent to a navicular score of 19 (MacGregor, 1984).
Similar changes were identified in the right front navicular
bone. Thus, the clinical and radiographic signs were compat-
ible with navicular disease, but this could not be confirmed
by local anaesthesia. Anaesthetic was not introduced into the
navicular bursa. The author has been unable to retrieve
synovial fluid from the bursa consistently and feels that a
negative response to anaesthesia is difficult to interpret,

although a positive response helps to confirm a diagnosis of navicular syndrome. The technique should be performed under radiographic control.

NECESSITY TO DESENSITIZE A LARGER AREA THAN ANTICIPATED FOR PROPOSED SITE OF LESION

Fracture of the distal phalanx

A 5-year-old polo pony had become acutely lame during a polo match and, despite 4 months box rest, had shown minimal improvement. The pony demonstrated moderate left forelimb lameness at walk, which was accentuated as it turned and was more marked at trot. Flexion of the left interphalangeal joints did not alter the lameness.

Percussion and pressure applied to the feet with hoof testers did not cause pain. After palmar (abaxial sesamoid) nerve blocks, the lameness was unchanged. Palmar (mid cannon) and palmar metacarpal (base of splint) nerve blocks rendered the horse sound. No radiographic abnormality of the left metacarpophalangeal and proximal interphalangeal joints was detected. There was a slightly displaced articular fracture of the medial one third of the distal phalanx.

Fractures of the distal phalanx are not uncommon in polo ponies and the referring clinician had suspected this injury at the time of onset of lameness. Because anaesthesia of the foot had not improved the lameness, a radiographic examination of the foot had not been performed. Post mortem examination revealed no significant pathology, other than the fracture described. The distribution of the nerves appeared normal, thus it is not clear why apparent desensitization of the foot failed to improve the lameness.

Fracture of the navicular bone

A 7-year-old pleasure horse had shown intermittent, mild right forelimb lameness since purchase 6 months previously. Compared to the left front foot the right front foot was more upright and narrow. The medial heel of the right front foot was higher than the lateral heel. There was a horny proliferative mass on the palmar medial aspect of the heel and pastern. Mild right forelimb lameness was apparent at walk and trot, and was accentuated if the horse turned sharply to the right. The lameness was most obvious on a hard surface.

Regional anaesthesia distal to the carpus did not improve the lameness. The horse was sound after median and ulnar nerve blocks. No radiographic abnormality of the right carpus, metacarpal, fetlock and pastern regions was detected. There was a slightly displaced fracture through the medial one third of the navicular bone, with radiolucent areas in the bone adjacent to the fracture line, and along the distal border of the navicular bone. No radiographic abnormality of the left navicular bone was detected.

This horse demonstrated clinical signs suggestive of a foot problem, but was rendered sound only by desensitization of the entire limb, distal to the elbow. The only radiographic abnormality was a displaced fracture of the navicular bone. The possibility of concurrent damage of the navicular bursa and deep digital flexor tendon cannot be excluded. Complete desensitization of the deep digital flexor tendon within the foot may require regional anaesthesia proximal to the carpus.

More than one cause of lameness

A 2-year-old thoroughbred colt exhibited moderate left fore-limb lameness of several weeks duration. There was a small, firm swelling over the proximal one third of the second metacarpal bone (a "splint") and pressure applied to it caused pain. Lameness was improved but not alleviated by infiltration of a local anaesthetic around the swelling. A palmar (abaxial sesamoid) nerve block did not alter the lameness. Palmar (mid cannon, distal to the "splint") and palmar metacarpal (base of splint) nerve blocks improved the lameness. If these nerve blocks were combined with infiltration of local anaesthetic around the described swelling the horse was sound. Radiographic examination revealed a subchondral bone cyst in the medial condyle of the third metacarpal bone and an active periosteal reaction on the proximal one third of the second metacarpal bone. Both of these lesions were considered to contribute to lameness. Without the use of local anaesthesia it would have been assumed that the "splint" was the only cause of lameness.

INTRA-ARTICULAR ANAESTHESIA

LAMENESS ASSOCIATED WITH A JOINT, RELIEVED BY REGIONAL ANAESTHESIA, BUT UNAFFECTED BY INTRA-ARTICULAR ANAESTHESIA

Presumed periarticular pathology

A 7-year-old thoroughbred showjumper had been lame on the left hindlimb for several months. Box rest resulted in some improvement, but lameness recurred when regular work was resumed. There was moderate thickening of the left hind metatarsophalangeal (fetlock) joint capsule, but the joint capsule did not feel distended. Passive flexion of the joint was not resented. The effect of flexion tests on the lameness was difficult to assess, because of the horse's temperament.

Regional anaesthesia of the foot did not improve the lameness, but plantar (mid cannon) and plantar metatarsal (base of splint) nerve blocks substantially improved the lameness.

The lameness was unaffected by subsequent intra-articular anaesthesia of the metatarsophalangeal joint. No significant radiographic abnormality was detected. It was assumed that the pain was periarticular, originating from soft tissue structures, e.g. joint capsule, collateral ligaments. The horse received an additional 3 months rest, and has been in regular work and sound for 6 months at the time of writing.

Enlargement of the fetlock joint capsule may be the result of distension by excessive synovial fluid, which may reflect significant intra-articular pathology. Alternatively, the enlargement may be the result of thickening of the capsule itself, and reflect primary periarticular pathology. In the latter case intra-articular anaesthesia is unlikely to improve the lameness.

Periarticular fibrosis

A 6-year-old pony had originally presented with a dislocation of the right scapulohumeral joint which had been successfully reduced with the pony under general anaesthesia. Six months later mild lameness persisted and although no radiographic abnormality of the joint was detected, pathology secondary to the dislocation was suspected.

Intra-articular anaesthesia did not improve the lameness, but during insertion of the needle, it could be appreciated that the periarticular soft tissues were firmer and more resistant than usual, probably because of fibrosis, and it was considered that the latter caused lameness. The pony resumed work despite mild lameness, progressively improved and is now sound.

Pathology of a proximal sesamoid bone

A 4-year-old thoroughbred racehorse had been intermittently lame for several months, and short periods of rest produced temporary improvement only. There was moderate thickening of the right metatarsophalangeal joint capsule, especially in the region of the proximal out-pouching. Distension of the joint capsule could not be appreciated. The medial and lateral branches of the suspensory ligament felt normal. Passive flexion of the joint was not resented, but accentuated the right hindlimb lameness.

Neither desensitization of the foot, nor intra-articular anaesthesia of the metatarsophalangeal joint, affected the lameness, which was relieved by plantar (mid cannon) and plantar metatarsal (base of splint) nerve blocks. Radiographic examination revealed a linear radiopacity proximal to and contiguous with the lateral proximal sesamoid bone, and a small, non-displaced apical fracture of the bone. These were probably associated with damage of the lateral branch of the suspensory ligament. Ultrasonography was not performed.

Although the proximal sesamoid bones are within the joint capsule, some of the aforementioned pathology was probably extracapsular.

Severe intra-articular pathology

A 6-year-old thoroughbred had exhibited left hindlimb lameness for 6 months and had shown no improvement, despite rest. There was slight distension of the left femoropatellar joint and flexibility of the limb was restricted. Holding the leg out behind the horse, without flexing the hock, accentuated the lameness. Flexion of the hip, stifle and hock joints caused a more marked exacerbation of the lameness.

Intra-articular anaesthesia of each of the femoropatellar, lateral and medial femorotibial joints, all performed within 1 h, did not alter the lameness. Radiographic examination of the stifle revealed flattening and remodelling of the medial femoral condyle and an osteophyte on the proximomedial aspect of the tibia at the distal site of attachment of the collateral ligament of the femorotibial joint.

Post mortem examination revealed no gross periarticular pathology, but extensive degenerative changes involving the medial femorotibial joint. Presumably such severe degenerative changes are associated with subchondral pain which is not relieved by intra-articular anaesthesia.

DISCUSSION

Although regional and intra-articular anaesthesia are invaluable techniques facilitating lameness diagnosis, it is important to be aware of their limitations, as illustrated by the cases described above. In a series of 250 horses investigated by the author there were difficulties in interpreting the results in approximately 5%.

Neither technique is a substitute for a thorough clinical examination. It is important to consider the results of anaesthesia in the light of clinical observations and to select appropriate areas for radiographic and, or, ultrasonic examination accordingly.

EFFECTIVE DESENSITIZATION

In the majority of horses, if effective desensitization of a region is achieved and the horse remains lame, then pain originates proximal to the site of injection. Effective desensitization may be difficult to assess especially in stoical horses. Cutaneous desensitization is not always synonymous with loss of deep sensation and vice versa.

There is some individual variation in nerve distribution, e.g. there may be an accessory branch (or branches) of the palmar digital nerve which arises proximal to the usual site for a palmar digital nerve block and transmits deep sensation from the palmar (caudal) aspect of the foot. Thus there may be cutaneous desensitization without relief of lameness despite originating in the palmar aspect of the foot.

In the hindleg, the dorsal metatarsal III nerve provides some cutaneous innervation to the dorsal aspect of the pastern region, therefore a plantar (abaxial sesamoid) nerve block will not necessarily remove all cutaneous sensation from this area (Wheat and Jones, 1981), but it should relieve pain originating in the foot.

Although median and ulnar nerve blocks should alleviate lameness associated with deep pain in the carpus or distally, the only areas which receive cutaneous innervation from these nerves only are the medial aspect of the pastern and the dorsolateral aspects of the metacarpal region. Other areas usually retain cutaneous sensation (Dyson, 1984).

DEGREE OF IMPROVEMENT

Some conditions, particularly those causing severe pain, e.g. pus in the foot, laminitis, may only be partially improved by regional anaesthesia. Conditions causing less severe pain are usually improved substantially by regional anaesthesia, although the horse may not be sound. A moderate improvement only may indicate multifocal causes of lameness, requiring further investigation. It can be difficult to decide whether or not a sufficient improvement has been made. It is helpful to assess the horse moving on hard and soft surfaces, in straight lines and in circles, in hand and ridden. There may be both painful and mechanical components to lameness in which case local anaesthesia would not be expected to relieve the lameness completely.

SLIGHT OR INTERMITTENT LAMENESS

In horses which are only slightly lame, assessment of improvement can be extremely difficult without the aid of sophisticated gait analysis equipment. It is hard to assess the effect of local anaesthesia, especially if the lameness is intermittent, unless the horse is rendered sound.

Every effort should be made to observe the horse moving under the conditions in which the lameness is most obvious, e.g. ridden with the rider sitting on either the left or right diagonal. Some time should be spent observing the horse before anaesthesia to ensure that the horse does not improve spontaneously with work.

JOINT PAIN

Joint pain is primarily the result of deep pressure caused by joint capsule distension, synovial fluid effusions and vascular engorgement especially of bone (Fessler, 1984). Synovial membrane inflammation and subchondral bone injuries also contribute to pain.

The joint capsule and collateral ligaments are richly inner- vated receiving articular branches from main nerve trunks, muscular branches and cutaneous branches. Periosteal branches supply the periosteum and perichondrium both of which are continuous with the joint capsule attachments to bone. The synovial membrane is less well innervated. Endo- steal branches which enter the bone marrow via the nutrient foramen innervate subchondral bone and these branches may preclude the complete desensitization of a joint by regional anaesthesia. Articular cartilage is not innervated. Intra- articular anaesthesia may alleviate pain associated with the synovial membrane but is unlikely to remove totally pain associated with the joint capsule and collateral ligaments and their attachments to bone, or pain from the subchondral bone.

INTRA-ARTICULAR ANAESTHESIA

In the cases described in this report in which intra-articular anaesthesia was employed, synovial fluid was always retrieved, thus confirming the intra-articular location of the needle. In the author's experience it is difficult to retrieve synovial fluid from the proximal interphalangeal (pastern) and the centrodistal (distal intertarsal) joints and it is necessary to rely on lack of resistance to injection of 4–6 ml of local anaesthetic. Similarly, unless the femoropatellar joint capsule is distended it is sometimes difficult to retrieve synovial fluid from the joint. The joint capsule bulges forward most cranially between the middle and medial patellar ligaments and this is the preferred site for injection.

In joints with severe intra-articular pathology, there may be minimal quantities of synovial fluid, so its retrieval is difficult. Intra-articular anaesthesia may not improve the lameness because of the extent and nature of the damage.

This report is not intended to be complete, nor to discourage the use of regional and intra-articular anaesthesia. The cases described represent only a small proportion of horses in which local anaesthesia has been usefully employed. The report does not try to explain why, in some circumstances, the results of a detailed clinical examination and local anaesthesia do not concur. It does emphasize the need for an accurate history, a careful clinical assessment and some of the limitations of the diagnostic techniques available. It also illustrates how, with experience, relevant information can be gained when inserting a needle before injection of local anaesthetic, even if the local anaesthetic does not improve the lameness.

ACKNOWLEDGEMENT

Mrs M. Cole is thanked for typing the manuscript.

REFERENCES

Colbern, G. (1984). *Compendium Continuing Education* 6, S611.
Dyson, S. (1984). *Veterinary Record* Supplement *In Practice* 6, 102.

Fessler, J. (1984). *Textbook of Large Animal Surgery* (ed. P. Jennings), p.687. Philadelphia, W. B Saunders.

MacGregor, C. (1984). PhD thesis.

Wheat, J. & Jones, K. (1981). *Veterinary Clinics North America: Large Animal Practice* **3**, 223.

CHAPTER 16

Variations in the Normal Radiographic Anatomy of Equine Limbs

SUSAN J. DYSON

INTRODUCTION

Radiography is an integral part of the investigative procedure for the evaluation of a lame horse and is being used increasingly as part of a pre-purchase examination, but interpretation of the radiographs is not always straightforward. The importance of good quality radiographs and a complete radiographic study of the area being examined cannot be over emphasized. Even with these it is sometimes difficult to assess the clinical significance of a lesion and a normal anatomical feature can easily be misinterpreted as a potential cause of lameness. This chapter describes some of the variations in radiographic anatomy which may be encountered in normal horses, free from lameness, and which are not necessarily of clinical significance. Discussion is restricted to the skeletally mature horse, serves as a guideline only and is by no means complete.

The anatomical nomenclature used in this article complies with Nomina Anatomica Veterinaria (1983) but colloquial names are mentioned in parentheses to facilitate understanding. The radiographic projections are described using the methods recommended by the American College of Veterinary Radiology and outlined by Smallwood and others (1985).

Radiographic interpretation can be facilitated by comparing

each radiograph with an equivalent bone specimen and with a reference radiograph of a clinically normal horse of similar age and type. If doubt about the significance of an abnormality persists it can often be helpful to obtain a similar view of the contralateral limb of the same horse.

This is not the place to describe radiographic techniques in detail, but there are several comments pertinent to this discussion. In some circumstances it can be useful to look at the area under suspicion using a different radiographic projection. For example the navicular bone can be assessed using not only lateromedial and dorso 60° proximal-palmaro-distal oblique (D60° Pr-PaDiO) or the "upright pedal, high coronary" views but also dorsopalmar (DPa) or dorso 30° proximal-palmarodistal oblique (D30° Pr-PaDiO) and palmaro-proximal-palmarodistal oblique (PaPr-PaDiO) views (Fig. 16.1). Slight variations in either exposure factors or obliquity of the X-ray beam may be helpful to define a suspicious area better.

The following comments concerning the distal forelimbs may also be applied to the hindlimbs.

DISTAL (THIRD) PHALANX (COFFIN OR PEDAL BONE)

The solar margin of the distal phalanx, as assessed in a dorso 60° proximal-palmarodistal projection, is usually regular and smooth (Fig. 16.2) but at the toe there may be a variably sized V-shaped notch, the crena marginis solearis (Fig. 16.3). It is usually similar in size and shape in both fore feet. In some older horses the outline of the solar margin may be slightly irregular (Fig. 16.4). The trabecular pattern of the distal phalanx is usually uniform and is divided by radially orientated vascular channels of variable width. Relatively broad vascular channels, or those that get wider closer to the margin of the distal phalanx may be seen in normal horses (compare Figs 16.2, 16.3 and 16.4).

Some degree of mineralization or ossification of the cartilages of the foot (side bone) occurs commonly, especially in hunters and heavier types of horse. It may occur symmetrically or involve only the medial or the lateral cartilage (Fig. 16.2). The latter may reflect chronic imbalance of the foot but is not

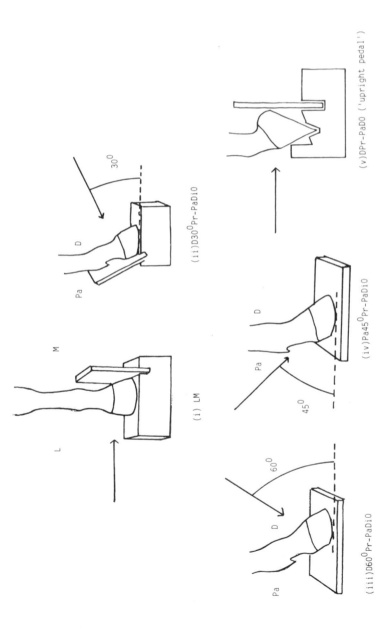

Fig. 16.1 Standard views of the foot. (i) Lateromedial (LM), (ii) Dorso 30° proximal-palmarodistal oblique (D30° Pr-PaDiO), (iii) Dorso 60° proximal-palmarodistal oblique (D60°-PaDiO). (iv) Palmaro 45° proximal-palmarodistal oblique (Pa45° Pr-PaDiO), (v) Dorsoproximal-palmarodistal oblique ("upright pedal" view), an alternative to (iii) D Dorsal. Pa Palmar. Pr Proximal. Di Distal. L Lateral. M Medial. O = oblique.

(i) LM

(ii)D30⁰Pr-PaDiO

(iii)D60⁰Pr-PaDiO

(iv)Pa45⁰Pr-PaDiO

(v)DPr-PaDO ('upright pedal')

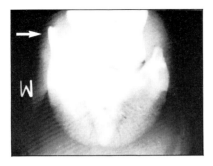

Fig. 16.2
D60 Pr-PaDiO view of a fore foot. There is
ossification of the medial cartilage of the foot
(arrow). The solar margin of the distal phalanx is
regular.

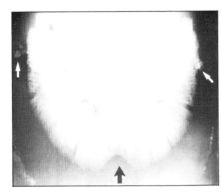

Fig. 16.3
D60 Pr-PaDiO view of a fore foot. There is a large
V-shaped notch, the crena marginis solearis, at the
toe of the distal phalanx (large arrow). The vascular
channels are broad. There is some mud on or in
the foot (small arrows).

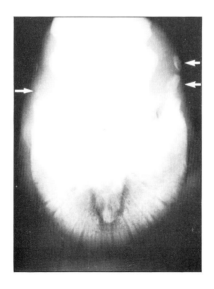

Fig. 16.4
D60 Pr-PaDiO view of a fore foot. The cartilages of
the foot are ossified in separate centres (arrows).

necessarily associated with lameness. The cartilage may ossify from separate centres of ossification (Fig. 16.4) resulting in discrete "islands" of bone. The intervening radiolucent lines should not be misinterpreted as fractures. The extent of ossification of the cartilages of the foot may be exaggerated in a dorso 60° proximal-palmarodistal oblique view and is more accurately assessed in either a dorsopalmar view or a dorso 30° proximal-palmarodistal oblique view.

The contour of the extensor process of the distal phalanx is smooth but it may have a single or double prominence, and be of variable size (Fig. 16.5a,b,c). Occasionally the extensor process has a smoothly rounded bony radiopacity proximal to it (Fig. 16.6) which occurs unilaterally or bilaterally. The contour of the extensor process appears normal. This may be a separate centre of ossification, an old chip fracture or ossification in the extensor tendon. In association with a recent chip fracture there is often some irregularity in outline of the extensor process. However, in

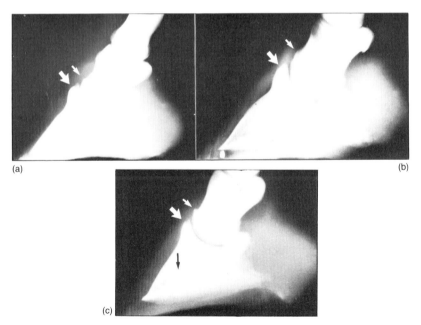

(a)

(b)

(c)

Fig. 16.5 LM views of three fore feet showing the variation in contour of the extensor process of the distal phalanx (large white arrows) and the distal dorsal aspect of the middle phalanx (small white arrows). The solar canal is seen end-on in 16.5c.

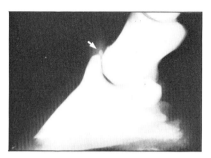

Fig. 16.6
LM view of a fore foot. There is a separate bone piece on the proximal aspect of the extensor process of the distal phalanx (arrow), either a separate centre of ossification, an ectopic centre of ossification or an old chip fracture.

some horses it may be difficult to discriminate radiographically between a fracture and a separate centre of ossification. The clinical significance of such a lesion in a lame horse is best assessed by intra-articular anaesthesia of the distal interphalangeal joint.

In a lateromedial projection the solar canal of the distal phalanx is seen end-on with a variable degree of clarity (Fig. 16.5c). It sometimes appears as a very distinct radiolucent zone in the middle of the bone proximal to the solar surface. The ease with which this is seen depends on the exposure factors used and the direction of the X-ray beam. It should not be confused with an osseous cyst-like lesion.

It must be remembered that slight obliquity of the X-ray beam will alter the apparent shape of normal structures. For a lateromedial projection of the foot the X-ray beam should be parallel to a line tangential to the horse's heels and should be centred on the area of interest; a divergent X-ray beam can also alter the contour of a normal structure. Appropriate preparation of the foot prior to radiography is essential to avoid confusing artefacts. Mud on or in the foot can mimic a bony radiopacity (Fig. 16.3).

SUMMARY OF STANDARDIZED NOMENCLATURE FOR RADIOGRAPHIC PROJECTIONS OF THE LIMBS (TABLE 16.1)

Table 16.1 Standardized nomenclature for radiographic projections of the limbs.

Name of projection	Abbreviation	Previously used equivalent term
Proximal to the antebrachiocarpal and tarsocrural joints		
Craniocaudal	CrCd	Anteroposterior
Caudocranial	CdCr	Posteroanterior
Craniolateral-caudomedial oblique	CrL-CdMO	Anteroposterior-lateromedial oblique
Craniomedial-caudolateral oblique	CrM-CdLO	Anteroposterior-mediolateral oblique
Carpus and tarsus and more distal limb		
Dorsopalmar	DPa	Anteroposterior
Dorsoplantar	DPl	Anteroposterior
Dorsolateral-palmaromedial oblique	DL-PaMO	Anteroposterior-lateromedial oblique
Dorsomedial-palmarolateral oblique	DM-PaLO	Anteroposterior-mediolateral oblique

DISTAL SESAMOID (NAVICULAR) BONE

In a dorso 60° proximal-palmarodistal oblique view the proximal border of the navicular bone may look irregular (Fig. 16.7) due to the obliquity of the X-ray beam. This border is assessed better in a dorsopalmar view. An entheseophyte is new bone at the site of a ligamentous insertion. New bone along the proximal border or on the medial or lateral proximal margins represents entheseophytes at the attachment of the collateral (suspensory) ligaments of the navicular bone. Although these may be associated with lameness they are not necessarily so. The distal border of the navicular bone can only be assessed properly if it is projected proximal to the distal interphalangeal joint. Several radiolucent areas, approximately triangular in shape, may be seen along the distal border of the navicular

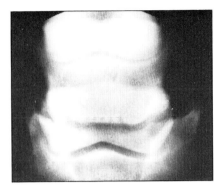

Fig. 16.7
D60 Pr-PaDiO view of a front foot. The proximal border of the navicular bone appears slightly irregular. There are at least five small radiolucent zones along the distal border of the navicular bone. The foot had been packed with PlayDoh but the frog cleft was not filled completely and the vertical radiolucent line through the middle phalanx represents this.

bone (Fig. 16.7). These represent synovial fossae and nutrient foramina which are not necessarily abnormal. There may be slightly sclerotic bone proximal to these radiolucent areas.

If the cleft of the frog and the medial and lateral sulci of the foot are not packed with a suitable radiopaque material such as PlayDoh there may be confusing radiolucent line(s) traversing the navicular bone which can mimic a fracture (Fig. 16.8). A radiolucent area may appear within the navicular bone which resembles a cystic lesion within the bone. If there is any doubt as to whether the "lesions" are real or artefacts, the radiograph is scrutinized to determine whether the radiolucent line extends beyond the margin of the bone. If there is a radiolucent area within the bone its position relative to the borders of the bone is measured carefully and compared with

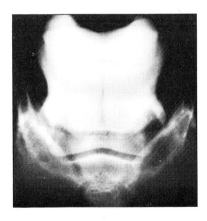

Fig. 16.8
D60 Pr-PaDiO view of a front foot. There is a radiolucent line through the centre of the navicular bone, which extends beyond the proximal border of the bone. This line, which mimics a fracture, is the shadow of the frog cleft.

a similar view obtained with a slightly different angle of the X-ray beam. An artefact will move relative to the margins of the bone. Dorsopalmar and palmaroproximal-palmarodistal oblique views are also useful to confirm whether such suspect lesions are real because in these projections the frog is not superimposed over the bone.

MIDDLE (SECOND) PHALANX (SHORT PASTERN BONE)

The contour of the distal dorsal aspect of the middle phalanx in a lateromedial projection is variable. It may be smoothly rounded (Figs. 16.5a,b) or have a sharp prominence (Fig. 16.5c) (which is exaggerated in a slightly oblique lateromedial view). The latter represents the dorsal limit of the distal articular surface of the middle phalanx. Proximal to this there may be a smoothly outlined bony prominence, the site of attachment of the collateral ligament of the distal interphalangeal joint. This may be variable in size and is again enhanced in a slightly oblique view and is most obvious in hunters and heavier types of horses. A small medullary cavity is occasionally present in this bone. It is usually spherical and should not be confused with a cyst-like lesion. It is easily superimposed over the navicular bone in dorsoproximal-palmarodistal oblique views, mimicking a radiolucent lesion in the navicular bone.

PROXIMAL (FIRST) PHALANX (LONG PASTERN BONE)

The medullary cavity is sometimes seen as a distinct radiolucency, approximately 2–3 cm in diameter, in the centre of the distal one half of the proximal phalanx (Fig. 16.9). In other horses the medullary cavity is barely distinguishable from the surrounding trabecular bone (Fig. 16.10). Occasionally a discrete radiolucent line within the centre of the bone is seen in either dorsopalmar or slightly oblique views (Fig. 16.10a, b). This must not be confused with a fissure fracture. The ergot is often superimposed over the proximal aspect of the proximal phalanx resulting in a round bony radiopacity (Fig.

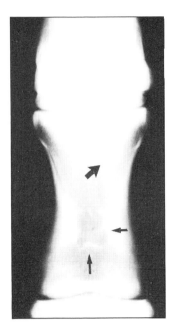

Fig. 16.9
DPa view of the proximal phalanx. The large radiolucent zone in the distal one-half of the bone (small arrows) represents the medullary cavity. The ergot is seen as a circular area of increased radiopacity (large arrow) on the proximal aspect of the bone.

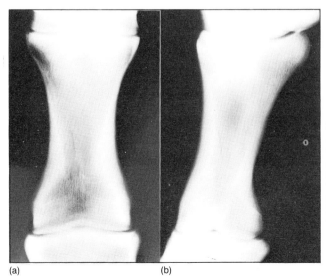

(a)   (b)

Fig. 16.10
DPa and DL-PaMO views of the proximal phalanx showing a radiolucent line within the bone which is probably an interoscos blood vessel.

16.9). New bone (entheseophytes) on the palmar medial and or palmar lateral aspects of the middle of the proximal phalanx occurs commonly, at the sites of insertion of the middle distal sesamoidean ligaments (Fig. 16.11). The bone may be smooth in outline or slightly irregular and variable in amount. It is of unlikely clinical significance unless it has a fuzzy outline or is accompanied by considerable calcification in the soft tissues on the palmar aspect of the proximal phalanx. Nevertheless a careful clinical examination of the area is warranted and possibly ultrasonographic examination of the distal sesamoidean ligaments.

Smoothly rounded extra-articular bony fragments are occasionally seen on the palmar aspect of the lateral or medial tuberosities of the proximal palmar aspect of the proximal phalanx. These may represent old fractures but are rarely associated with lameness.

METACARPOPHALANGEAL/METATARSOPHALANGEAL (FETLOCK) JOINT

In some horses there is slight remodelling of the dorsal aspects of the proximal phalanx, highlighted in oblique views (Fig.

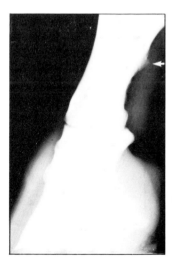

Fig. 16.11
DL-PaMO view of the phalanges. There is an irregularly, but smoothly, outlined bony eminence on the palmar lateral aspect of the proximal phalanx (arrow), an entheseophyte at the site of insertion of the middle distal sesamoidean ligament.

16.12). Small osteophytes disrupt the normally smoothly curved contour of the dorsoproximal aspect of the proximal phalanx. Such changes may reflect degenerative joint disease but do not necessarily do so and their significance must be interpreted in the light of the clinical signs. This is often seen in horses of middle age or older, especially common types.

Small separate bony radiopacities on the dorsoproximal aspect of the proximal phalanx can occur unilaterally or bilaterally (Fig. 16.13). They are usually smoothly rounded and the contour of the dorsoproximal aspect of the proximal phalanx appears regular. They may be attached by fibrous tissue to the proximal phalanx and thus move with it; therefore in a flexed lateral view they remain in the same position relative to the proximal phalanx. These may be separate centres of ossification, ectopic ossification or old chip fractures. With some chip fractures the area from which the fracture arose can be detected radiographically. The radiographs must be interpreted with reference to the clinical signs; small, clinically significant, chip fractures are usually accompanied by distension of the joint capsule and some pain on passive flexion of the joint.

Assessment of the width of the joint space in the dorsopalmar view is only possible if the proximal sesamoid bones are projected proximally to the joint and this can be achieved by

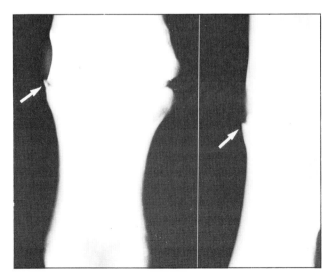

Fig. 16.12
Slightly oblique DPa and DL-PaMO views of the metacarpophalangeal joint. There is a small osteophyte on the dorsomedial aspect of the proximal phalanx (arrow).

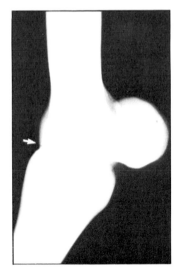

Fig. 16.13
LM view of the metacarpophalangeal joint. There is a separate
bone piece on the dorsoproximal aspect of the proximal
phalanx, either a separate centre of ossification, an ectopic
focus of ossification or an old chip fracture.

angling the X-ray beam from proximally to distally at least
10°. The X-ray beam must be centred approximately at the
level of the joint. A false impression of narrowing of the joint
space may be obtained if the X-ray beam is centred proximal
or distal to the joint.

SECOND, THIRD AND FOURTH METACARPAL/METATARSAL (SPLINT AND CANNON) BONES

In a dorsopalmar view the nutrient foramen of the third
metacarpal bone is seen end-on as a small radiolucent area at
the junction between the proximal and middle one-thirds of
the bone. In a lateral view this may be seen as an oblique
radiolucent line which should not be confused with a fracture
of either the cortex of the third metacarpal bone or the
second or fourth metacarpal bones, across which it may be
superimposed (Fig. 16.14).

In a lateromedial view there is superimposition of the
second, third and fourth metacarpal bones and this may result
in vertically orientated radiolucent lines in the second or
fourth metacarpal bones which should not be misinterpreted
as fractures. In some horses a radiolucent line extends distally

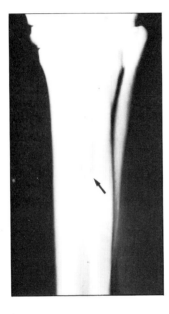

Fig. 16.14
DL-PIMO view of the metatarsus. The nutrient foramen of the
third metatarsus is superimposed over the second metatarsal
bone resulting in a radiolucent line that mimics a fracture
(arrow).

from the medullary cavity in the proximal part of either the
second or fourth metacarpal bones; it finishes on the dorsal
aspect of the bone in its middle one-third and probably
represents a nutrient artery (Fig. 16.15). These lines occur
unilaterally or bilaterally.

Ossification between the second and or fourth metacarpal
bones and the third metacarpal bone occurs commonly in a
localized area (Fig. 16.16) or, more rarely, extends throughout
their lengths (Fig. 16.17). In many horses there is even or
irregular, but smoothly outlined, new bone on the second or
fourth metacarpal bones, the result of previous trauma to the
bone. This should be distinguished from an active periosteal
reaction which has an indistinct or fuzzy outline. The accumulation of new bone around either the second or fourth
metacarpal bones may result in obliquely orientated radiolucent lines through the bones which must not be confused
with fractures. The distal ends of the second and fourth
metacarpal bones are variable both in their size and shape
and distance from the third metacarpal bone.

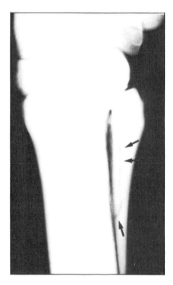

Fig. 16.15
DL-PaMO view of the metacarpus. There is a radiolucent line in the proximal one-half of the fourth metacarpal bone (arrows).

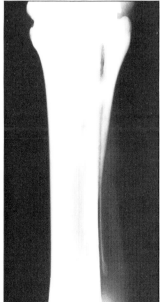

Fig. 16.16
DL-PaMO view of the metacarpus. There is partial ossification between the third and fourth metacarpal bones.

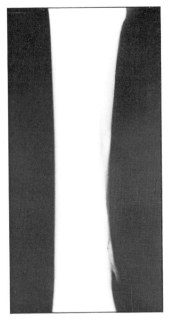

Fig. 16.17
DM-PaMO view of the metacarpus. The second and third
metacarpal bones are fused.

CARPUS

The carpus is a complex structure and in all views the carpal
bones are partially superimposed over each other. This results
in some confusing radiolucent lines which should not be
mistaken for fractures.

The first and fifth carpal bones may be present or absent at
the level of the carpometacarpal joint (Fig. 16.18). Occasionally
there is an extra small bone at the level of the intercarpal joint.
A first carpal bone is present more frequently than a fifth
carpal bone, and may be partially superimposed over the
second carpal bone in all views. An irregular radiolucent area
may be seen within either or both of the first or second carpal
bones (Fig. 16.19). Cystic lesions also occur in the second
carpal bones without a first carpal bone being present and in
any of the other carpal bones (Fig. 16.20). They are frequently
of no significance but a large lesion close to an articular surface
may be a cause of lameness.

Periosteal proliferative reactions on the dorsal aspects of the
carpal bones, especially the radial and third carpal bones,

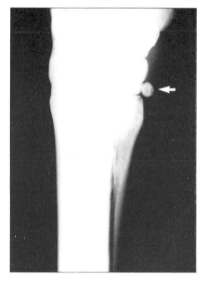

Fig. 16.18
DM-PaLO view of the carpus. There is a first carpal bone.

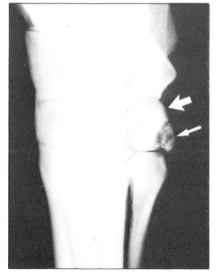

Fig. 16.19
DM-PaLO view of a carpus. The first carpal bone (small arrow) is partially superimposed over the second carpal bone (large arrow) and there are irregular radiolucent areas within each bone.

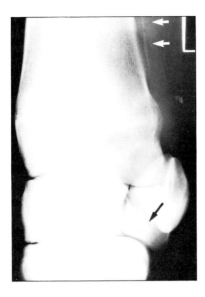

Fig. 16.20
DL-PaMO view of a carpus. There is a radiolucent osseous cyst-like lesion in the distal aspect of the ulnar carpal bone, which is surrounded by more sclerotic bone (black arrow). There is a vestigial ulna ossified in separate pieces.

occur at the sites of insertion of the intercarpal ligaments (Fig. 16.21). These periosteal reactions are seen most commonly in thoroughbreds which raced at two or three years of age. They are not indicative of degenerative joint disease and are seldom

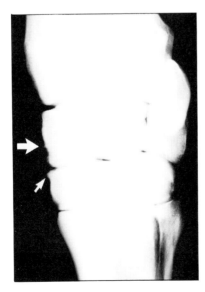

Fig. 16.21
DL-PaMO view of a carpus. There is periosteal new bone on the dorsomedial aspect of the radial carpal bone (large white arrow) of no significance, but there is a small osteophyte on the dorsomedial aspect of the third carpal bone (small white arrow) indicative of significant joint disease. There is a vestigial ulna which is not united to the radius.

of clinical significance, but do reflect a previous injury. The articular margins of the bones should nevertheless be inspected carefully and any irregularity probably indicates significant intra-articular disease.

ANTEBRACHIUM (FOREARM)

The transverse crest on the distal caudal aspect of the radius is variable in size and may be slightly irregular in outline with some fuzziness (Fig. 16.22). Proximal to this there may be a small bony eminence projecting from the caudal cortex of the radius and, if small, this is of no significance. Sometimes such exostoses are seen in association with distension of the carpal sheath and then they may be of clinical significance.

A vestigial ulna of variable size and shape is frequently present; it may or may not be united to the distal radius (Figs. 16.20, 16.21). The ulna is occasionally complete but is often incompletely ossified. The chestnut is seen approximately 10 cm proximal to the antebrachiocarpal joint and if partially superimposed over the radius may appear as a bony radiopacity.

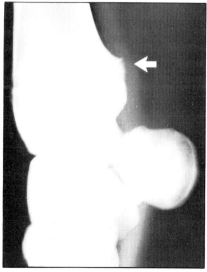

Fig. 16.22
LM view of a carpus. The proximal aspect of the transverse crest on the caudal aspect of the radius is irregular (arrow).

TARSUS (HOCK)

Clinically silent osteochondritic lesions are seen frequently in the tarsocrural (tibiotarsal) joint. The most common sites are the distal intermediate ridge of the tibia, the medial malleolus of the tibia and the distal end of the medial trochlear ridge of the talus (tibiotarsal bone). They appear as small discrete bony radiopacities. Although such lesions may be associated with distension of the tarsocrural joint capsule (bog spavin), lameness is unusual unless the pieces are very large.

The distal end of the medial trochlear ridge of the talus is extremely variable in shape and may be smoothly rounded, have a variably sized bony eminence or have a separate bony radiopacity distal to it (possibly an osteochrondritic lesion – see above) (Fig. 16.23a,b,c,d). Slight flattening of the medial and lateral trochlear ridges of the talus is not unusual.

Fusion of the centrodistal (distal intertarsal) and, or tarso-metatarsal joints is seen occasionally with no evidence of other bony lesions. A small osteophyte on the dorsoproximal aspect of the third metatarsal bone may be an entheseophyte at the site of attachment of the dorsal tarsometatarsal ligament, reflecting a previous injury, and, in the absence of other radiographic abnormalities, does not necessarily herald degenerative joint disease of the tarsometatarsal joint. It must be remembered that the chestnut of a hindlimb is projected at the level of the distal row of tarsal bones.

STIFLE

There is little variation in the normal radiographic anatomy of the stifle. The fibula may be short and vestigial, ossified in two or more centres or be complete (Figs 16.24a,b,c,d). The division between two separate centres of ossification must not be confused with a fracture. Slight flattening of the lateral trochlear ridge of the femur is sometimes seen; this is probably a subclinical manifestation of osteochondrosis. There may be slight sclerosis of the underlying subchondral bone. Sometimes the articular surface of the medial femoral condyle appears abnormally flat. A small dimple may occur in the middle of the

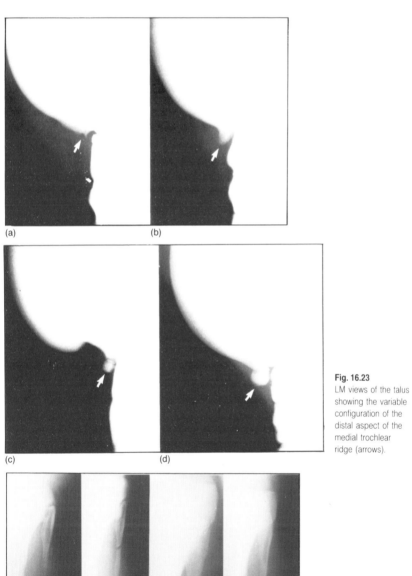

(a)   (b)

(c)   (d)

Fig. 16.23
LM views of the talus
showing the variable
configuration of the
distal aspect of the
medial trochlear
ridge (arrows).

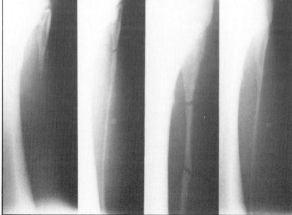

(a)   (b)   (c)   (d)

Fig. 16.24
CdCr views of the
stifle showing the
variable shapes and
degree of ossification
of the fibula.

articular surface and, although this may be clinically innocuous, occasionally a subchondral bone cyst develops at that site. Rarely, one or two discrete bony radiopacities are seen on the distal caudal aspect of the femur proximal to the condyles; these are fabellae.

CONCLUSIONS

There is considerable variation in the normal radiographic anatomy of the equine limbs, which is in part related to the age of the horse, its type and occupation and any previous injuries (clinical or subclinical). For example small periarticular osteophytes are often seen in older horses, but are more cause for concern in a young horse. Osteophytes may be the only radiographic abnormality detectable in association with degenerative joint disease, however their presence does not imply necessarily that the joint has ongoing intra-articular disease. Their significance must be interpreted with care. Entheseophytes (new bone at the site of ligamentous attachments) may reflect a previous injury, but are often not of long term significance.

It must be admitted that there is still a lack of knowledge concerning the potential importance to a horse of specific abnormalities, both in the immediate future and the long term. Ideally a large group of horses needs to be monitored both radiographically and clinically throughout their working lives so that a more objective assessment of the significance of some of the variations in radiographic anatomy can be made.

REFERENCES

Nomina Anatomica Veterinaria (1983). 3rd edn. New York, Ithaca. World Association of Veterinary Anatomists.
Smallwood, J., Shively, M., Rendano, V. & Habel, R. (1985). *Veterinary Radiology* **26**, 2.

CHAPTER 17

Equine Rhabdomyolysis Syndrome

PATRICIA A. HARRIS

INTRODUCTION

Tying-up, set fast and azoturia, etc. (see Table 17.1) may all be names used to describe variations in the clinical picture of the same syndrome. The term equine rhabdomyolysis has recently been used to encompass these various conditions, which primarily affect the musculature of horses.

Although such non-traumatic muscle myopathies have been well recognized for over 100 years, there has been little advancement in our understanding of the underlying biochemical lesion(s).

The epidemiology of this syndrome has changed over the years as the management and use of the horse has altered. For example, the classic "Monday morning" disease found primarily in the draught horse is not commonly seen, whereas

Table 17.1 Equine rhabdomyolysis syndrome: variations in the clinical picture

Tying-up	Exertional rhabdomyolysis
Set fast	Paralytic myoglobinuria
Azoturia	Monday morning disease
	Exertional myopathy

there appears to be an increased incidence in all types of performance horse.

The condition can occur at any age and in both sexes, although an increased incidence has been seen in young fillies. Many of the sufferers in this country are thoroughbred or thoroughbred crosses, which may reflect their high popularity at the present time for competitive riding. A familial predisposition has been suggested, but not confirmed.

CLINICAL SIGNS

The mildest form of this syndrome may present as a very slight stiffness or just a shortened stride; for example, a dressage or show pony may fail to lengthen when asked, or a racing animal may appear to fade towards the end of a race. The signs may range from a slight change in gait (often very difficult to distinguish from that caused by other conditions) to the more easily recognized reluctance or inability to move. In more severe cases recumbency and death can occur.

Often, in more severely affected animals, certain muscles may be hard, swollen and painful. Although it is usually the croup, loin and thigh muscles that are involved, cases have been seen where the forelimb(s), alone or in combination with other muscles, have been affected. In most cases there is bilateral involvement, but apparent unilateral cases have also been reported. Swelling or boarding of the muscles may not be apparent immediately. On occasions, pigmented urine due to the presence of myoglobin or its degradation products, is voided. However, this may not be pathognomonic for the syndrome.

The clinical signs are usually, but not always, triggered by exercise. They may be divided into five groups according to their severity as shown in Table 17.2. Some animals may show signs typical of more than one group.

ATYPICAL MYOGLOBINURIA

In this country, sudden death from the equine rhabdomyolysis syndrome is comparatively rare. However, workers at the Animal Health Trust and elsewhere have recently reported severe and often fatal attacks occurring in animals out at pasture, with no history of sudden exertion. This may, however, be a totally separate condition and has been referred to as atypical myoglobinuria. The outbreaks occurred mainly in Scotland, but isolated cases have also been reported in England and Wales. The main features of this condition are shown in Table 17.3.

DIAGNOSIS

The differential diagnosis of equine rhabdomyolysis should include the various conditions given in Table 17.4. It must be remembered that equine rhabdomyolysis may occur at the same time as other conditions such as "colic".

The diagnosis is usually made on the basis of the history, clinical picture and often laboratory investigations (Table 17.5). Electromyography and muscle biopsy are not commonly used for diagnosis in this country, however, these techniques may be of value in the future to help unravel the pathophysiology of this condition and perhaps enable a predisposition to be detected. More commonly, elevations of the enzyme creatine kinase (CK) and aspartate aminotransferase (AST) activities are used to confirm the diagnosis, give an indication of the severity and to monitor the recovery (Table 17.6).

Creatine kinase is found mainly in the skeletal muscle, but also, in significant amounts, in the heart and brain. It is rapidly cleared from the blood, having a half-life of around 2 h. After a single severe episode of muscle damage, the activity level peaks within 4–12 h and returns to normal within a few days if no further damage occurs. However, it must be noted that the level can increase slightly following unaccustomed exercise in the unfit horse and, even in the trained fit horse, increases can occur following strenuous exercise. Such increases may not represent actual damage to the muscle, but

Table 17.2 Grade of clinical severity.

Grade	Mobility	Muscle	Excessive sweating	Pulse and resp. rates elevated above expected levels	Signs normally attributed to GIT disturbances	Discoloured urine	Comments
I	Slight stiffness shortened stride	No abnormality detected	–	–	–	–	Easily confused with other conditions, often transient
II	Reluctant to move	Often no abnormality detected	±	+	±	–	Urine not usually discoloured
III	Unable to move	Firm swollen, resent palpation	+	+	+	+	
IV	Unable to move – may become transiently recumbent	Firm swollen, may not resent palpation	+ +	+ +	+ +	+ +	?palpation is actually felt by the horse
V	Rapidly become recumbent	Firm ± wasting	(+ +)	+ + +	+ + +	+ + +	GIT stasis can occur. Shock may develop. Death can occur

Table 17.3 Main features of atypical myoglobinuria.

Mainly horses/ponies out at grass.
Sudden onset of stiffness unrelated to exercise.
Animals are usually able to eat and drink normally.
Temperature, pulse rate and respiration rate are usually within normal range.
One or more animals within a group may be affected.
Dark, chocolate or blood coloured urine usually voided.
Markedly elevated creatine kinase activities.
Recumbency and death can occur.

Table 17.4 Possible differential diagnoses of equine rhabdomyolysis.

"Colic"
Iliac thrombosis
Laminitis
Tetanus
Castration sequelae
Damage to the spinal cord/nerve roots
Various "back" problems
Certain toxicities, e.g. acorn, monensin
Nutritionally-based myopathies
Certain neuromuscular disorders
Lyme disease (*Borrelia burgdorferi*)

Table 17.5 Laboratory aids for diagnosis.

Plasma/serum enzyme activities
Urinalysis
Electromyography
Muscle biopsy
(i) surgical (ii) needle
? Plasma electrolyte concentrations
? Acid–base status

Table 17.6 Use of plasma muscle enzyme activities.

AST (iu/l)	2000	6000	600	350	0-230
CK (iu/l)	8000	700	30	30	0- 50
Likely clinical stage	Active muscle damage early stages	Early recovery phase	Late recovery phase	?Late recovery or other soft tissue damage	Normal range*

*P. E. Burrell laboratory at AHT.

rather changes in the membrane permeability.

Aspartate aminotransferase is present in the mitochondria and cytosol of almost all cells, but mainly in the liver, heart and skeletal muscle. It is, therefore, not organ specific and there can be a significant rise with several forms of soft tissue damage. However, following an insult to the muscle, the AST activity of the plasma peaks about 24 h afterwards. The half-life is 7–8 days and the levels return to normal around 2–4 weeks later – if no further attacks occur (the time course obviously depends to some extent on the original extent of the rise in the activity). The level of plasma activity may increase slightly with exercise and in an individual may vary during training.

Lactate dehydrogenase (LDH) has also been used, but total LDH activity is not organ specific and the isoenzyme activities are more commonly used. These may be of particular value in detecting cases with cardiac involvement. LDH peaks around 12–24 h after an insult to the muscle and levels have been reported to return to normal within 5–10 days.

The difference in the respective half-life of these enzymes means that the relative activities can be used to determine the stage of muscle damage, i.e. active, early recovery or late recovery.

It has been suggested that the rise in activity is proportional to the degree of muscle fibre damage. However, the activities may not always reflect the severity of the clinical signs. Figure 17.1, for example, shows the CK levels from a Grade II and a Grade III severity case. As can be seen, far higher activities were recorded from the Grade II than the Grade III sufferer.

In addition, some animals that suffer from recurrent attacks

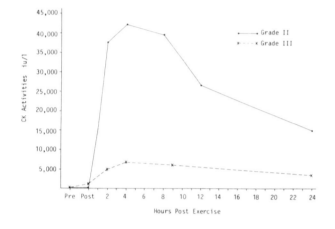

Fig. 17.1
CK activities (iu/l)
recorded for a
clinical Grade II and
Grade III severity
attack.

may show CK activities up to several thousand iu/litre without any obvious clinical signs. Others may show apparently typical signs without any marked elevation of CK and AST activities. This could be due to a misdiagnosis, or there may have been insufficient muscle mass damage to cause a significant rise in the enzyme activities (even though the damage to the muscle was sufficient to cause overt signs of pain). There may also be a separate condition with a completely different pathophysiology which can result in pure "spasm" of the muscles, rather than actual "damage".

Exercise tests may be of value for diagnosis especially of mild cases. However, the results must be interpreted with caution, allowing for the recent clinical history and fitness of the animal, as well as the intensity and duration of the exercise.

OTHER PARAMETERS

Measurement of serum electrolytes and blood acid-base status may be useful in more severe cases (as discussed below). In these cases, blood urea nitrogen and serum creatinine levels may also be of value in assessing the effects of dehydration and, or, myoglobin clearance on renal function.

PATHOPHYSIOLOGY

The pathophysiology of equine rhabdomyolysis is still obscure, although there have been numerous suggestions as to its cause (Table 17.7).

Carbohydrate overloading has been the most popular theory ever since Carlström (1932) reproduced the condition by exercising animals fed a high carbohydrate diet. However, this theory has recently been the subject of much debate. Work in racehorses has shown that the restoration of muscle glycogen, following depletion during exercise, takes several days. Therefore an occasional rest day would be unlikely to result in glycogen build-up. In addition, the actual increase in blood lactic acid found by Carlström (1932) and other workers is very small compared to that seen following racing. Cases of rhabdomyolysis are seen where alkalosis rather than acidosis occurs. It is, however, possible that there is just a local lactic acid build-up in a few fibres, which is not sufficient to cause an appreciable rise in blood levels.

Local hypoxia has been suggested as being important. However, if it is the only cause it is difficult to see how the condition can occur at light exercise when the low oxidative

Table 17.7 Possible predisposing causes of equine rhabdomyolysis.

(1) Faulty substrate metabolism
      Carbohydrate overloading
      Glycolytic enzyme deficiency
      Faulty fat metabolism
(2) Vitamin and mineral deficiencies
      Vitamin E and, or, selenium
      Thiamin
(3) Endocrine abnormalities
      Hypothyroidism
      Sex related
      Corticosteroid therapy
(4) Electrolyte imbalances
      Na^+, K^+, Ca^+, Mg^+, Ph^+
      Malignant hyperthermia
(5) Others
      Viral infections

fibres (predominantly affected in equine rhabdomyolysis), with their relatively poor capillary supply, have not even been recruited. It also does not explain why the condition is not usually seen in cases of aortic-iliac thrombosis.

In man, a myophosphorylase deficiency results in very similar clinical signs to those seen in equine rhabdomyolysis. However, human sufferers are usually unable to sustain any high intensity activity, which is unlike the intermittent equine condition. Deficiency of carnitine palmityl transferase (an enzyme involved in the breakdown of free fatty acids before they enter the Krebs cycle) can, in man, result in intermittent muscle stiffness and myoglobinuria. Unlike in equine rhabdomyolysis, the signs tend to occur after fasting and the respiratory muscles are often involved. Recent work investigating over 20 different muscle fibre enzymes could not establish a predisposition for equine rhabdomyolysis.

Although selenium/vitamin E deficiencies have been implicated in myopathies in various species, workers have found no evidence that selenium deficiency plays an important role in the majority of rhabdomyolysis cases.

Hypothyroidism is a common cause of myalgia in man and a limited study by Waldron-Mease (1979) suggested that equine rhabdomyolysis may be secondary to hypothyroidism. This author suggested that as cold, growth or non-specific stress increase the demands on the thyroid, the combined effects of training and such a superimposed stress may exceed the animal's capacity to respond with higher thyroxine output. Work is currently being carried out into this area at the Animal Health Trust. Hormonal differences between colts and fillies have been suggested as a reason for increased incidence in young fillies. However, results have shown no correlation between elevations in serum enzyme activities, or clinical manifestations of equine rhabdomyolysis and the stage of the oestrous cycle.

There are complex interactions between intracellular and extracellular ion concentrations and neuromuscular function. Disturbances in these ion concentrations may, therefore, affect the neuromuscular activity directly, or the resulting ionic imbalances may affect the cellular metabolism. The disturbance may be as a result of a simple dietary deficiency, or a more complicated absorptive/utilization problem. Work has recently been carried out at the Animal Health Trust into the possible role of calcium, phosphorous, sodium and potassium disturbances.

A similarity between equine rhabdomyolysis and the genetically influenced conditions of malignant hyperthermia in man and the porcine stress syndrome has been suggested and is discussed in more detail under prevention.

Myalgia or muscle cramping occurs after some viral infections in man and in the horse. Many owners and trainers have reported muscle stiffness occurring in their animals following a viral infection. However, this relationship has not been extensively studied or proven.

TREATMENT

The treatment can be divided into management and therapy.

MANAGEMENT

It is very difficult to distinguish between the muscle damage caused by the pathological condition of equine rhabdomyolysis and that caused by other non-traumatic myopathies, such as over-exertion, heat and electrolyte disturbances. Some mild cases of equine rhabdomyolysis and certain other conditions may respond to walking. For the majority, however, forced walking may exacerbate the muscle damage and increase the severity of the condition. Therefore, unless it is certain, for example, that mild over-exertion is the cause of the stiffness, it is usually advisable to give the affected animal immediate complete rest. In some cases even moving the horse home in a trailer can precipitate a much more severe attack.

The feed intake should, obviously, be reduced during this period of rest. In severe cases, just meadow hay, water and, if necessary, some low energy proprietary cubes should be fed. All cases should preferably be kept warm, dry and away from draughts in a well bedded area. Ideally, recumbent cases should not be forced to rise, but should be assisted to do so as soon as possible (all normal procedures for managing a recumbent case should be applied). In this condition, it is of particular importance to check that adequate urination occurs.

THERAPY

A list of some of the more commonly used therapeutic agents is given in Table 17.8, together with the general aims of such treatment (the dose rates for the more commonly used compounds are as recommended by the manufacturers).

In milder cases, analgesics are not always required and care should be taken when giving certain agents, especially if the attack of equine rhabdomyolysis is complicated by other disease processes. Care must also be taken with acepromazine and other phenothiazine derivatives due to their blocking action on the sympathetic nervous system, which can lead to hypovolaemia and shock. Corticosteroids may be of use in

Table 17.8 Therapeutic agents in the treatment of equine rhabdomyolysis.

Treatment aims to
    Limit further muscle damage
    Reduce pain and anxiety
    If necessary, restore fluid balance in order to maintain adequate
    kidney function

Therapeutic agents
(1) Analgesics
    (a) Phenylbutazone*
    (b) Flunixin meglumine*
    (c) Meclofenamic acid
    (d) Methadone if severely affected
(2) Sedatives/tranquillizers
    (a) Phenothiazine derivatives
    (b) Xylazine ⎱ especially in cases
                with a
    (c) Diazepam ⎰ compromised circulation
(3) Corticosteroids
    During the acute phase only
(4) Fluids
    (a) Very important
    (b) Not diuretics
(5) Others of doubtful value
    (a) Methocarbamol (muscle relaxant)
    (b) Dantrolene
    (c) Vitamin E/selenium
    (d) Thiamin
    (e) Sodium bicarbonate

*most commonly used

the initial acute stages as they perhaps stabilize cellular membranes and have been reported to produce relaxation of the capillary sphincters, which may help to improve tissue perfusion. Corticosteroid therapy itself, however, has been suggested to be a predisposing factor, but there is limited documentation on this. Recent work at the Animal Health Trust has not shown prior corticosteroid administration to be a factor in the history of equine rhabdomyolysis sufferers in the UK.

Due to uncertainty of the role of lactic acid in rhabdomyolysis and the fact that many cases show a metabolic alkalosis, rather than an acidosis, the rationale for the administration of sodium bicarbonate therapeutically has to be questioned, unless the acid-base status is known.

Although most workers in this field have found no correlation between vitamin E and selenium status and a predisposition to equine rhabdomyolysis, it has been suggested that they have some value in the treatment due to their action against tissue-damaging free radicals.

Fluid therapy is often essential. Oral fluids alone, such as half-strength Lectade (Beecham Animal Health) may be sufficient for the Grade III case. However, oral, plus intravenous, fluids are usually required for Grades IV and V. The amount and type of fluid that should be used depends to some extent on the nature of the exercise that preceded the attack. In most instances, balanced electrolyte solutions can be given, as with adequate kidney function the horse should be able to correct most acid-base and electrolyte disturbances. In severe cases, if possible, the acid-base and electrolyte status should be assessed and the animal treated accordingly. Clean water should be available for all cases.

It has been suggested that, if necessary, the fluid therapy should be maintained until the urine is free from pigmentation.

RETURN TO WORK

The speed at which an animal is returned to work depends on the severity of the episode and the animal's history. For example, it may be preferable in a recurrent sufferer, or an animal which has suffered a severe attack, to wait until both the AST and CK activities have returned to normal resting levels, whereas other animals may start working much earlier, once the CK activities are within acceptable limits.

Whenever possible, it is advisable to turn the horse out into a small paddock, after the period of box rest (the length of which depends on the clinical severity of the attack), before ridden exercise is given. Lungeing may not be advisable in the early stages of the return to work. Exercise should be increased gradually and the feed altered accordingly. Appropriate preventive measures should be taken. In recurrent sufferers an exercise test carried out after approximately 2 weeks may be of value.

PREVENTION

Prevention can be divided into the various management procedures that can be adopted and the prophylactic agents that can be used. Obviously, the basic rules of feeding a balanced diet and feeding according to the work being undertaken must be adhered to. A change in the exercise pattern has apparently been of value in some cases. This could involve daily exercise; twice daily exercise; longer warm-up periods; fewer short, fast spurts of exercise, but longer periods at a lower intensity, etc. Although procedures that are successful in one animal may not help another, the first preventive measure taken should be to ensure a well-balanced and controlled feeding and exercise regimen.

Prophylactically, many agents have been suggested over the years. Some of these are:

Vitamin E/selenium
Sodium bicarbonate
Dantrolene sodium
Thiamin
Thyroxine
Phenothiazine tranquillizers
Sodium salicylate
Dimethylglycine
Electrolytes

Bicarbonate may be of value in prevention, if a local lactic acidosis contributes to the muscle fibre damage. However, its efficacy in the prevention of equine rhabdomyolysis has not been scientifically proven.

Dantrolene has been used in human medicine to treat and help prevent malignant hyperthermia, which is an inherited myopathy that occurs on exposure to a triggering factor such as stress, excitement, anxiety, exercise or exposure to volatile anaesthetic agents and depolarizing muscle relaxants. In response to these factors, there is an abnormal release of calcium from the sarcoplasmic reticulum which results in a prolonged contracture. This in turn results in hyperthermia, metabolic and respiratory acidosis and muscle damage. Recently the halothane-caffeine contracture test used in man to diagnose this condition has been adapted for equine use. Using this test, some animals have been detected with contracture responses believed to be consistent with malignant hyperthermia. Dantrolene has been used to treat, but more usually to help prevent, further attacks of equine rhabdomyolysis, especially in the USA. Various doses have been used, such as 2 mg/kg once a day for 3–5 days (which may be continued by 2 mg/kg every third day for a month). However, it appears to be hepatotoxic and, as there are few reports of its beneficial use in the animal that has suffered repeated attacks of equine rhabdomyolysis, its true worth has been questioned.

Small doses of phenothiazine tranquillizers (e.g. acepromazine 0·01 mg/kg) given about 30 min before exercise have been suggested to help the "anxious" horse. However, care must be taken in their use, as they are prohibited substances. Recently, dimethylglycine (1 mg/kg orally) has been suggested to increase oxygen utilization, decrease blood lactate levels and reduce the incidence of equine rhabdomyolysis. At present, there is no scientific work to substantiate this claim, and the mechanism by which it acts is unclear. Therefore, at the moment, its use cannot be recommended.

Thyroxine (L-thyroxine sodium 0·1 mg/kg orally) has been recommended to improve exercise tolerance and to help sufferers of equine rhabdomyolysis.

Thiamin has been suggested as it aids in the breakdown of lactic acid and in the decarboxylation of pyruvic acid. Again, there is no scientific work to prove its efficacy.

Recent work at the Animal Health Trust has shown that correcting an electrolyte imbalance detected by a creatinine clearance test may help prevent further attacks in some animals: a prevention rate of approximately 60% has been found using such electrolyte supplementation. However, as with all such preventive measures, it has been difficult to prove true efficacy. This is firstly because the syndrome itself is intermittent and, therefore, it is not possible to determine if these animals would have suffered attacks if the supplementation had not been given; secondly, there are ethical problems of reproducing the condition, especially in referred clinical cases, by removing the apparently beneficial supplementation.

CONCLUSION

No single theory has been able to explain why this syndrome should occur in one animal, rather than others kept under identical managemental regimens. It appears that sufferers have an underlying abnormality that predisposes them to the condition and a triggering factor is then required to initiate the whole process, resulting in the clinical signs. The predisposing factor(s) and triggering factor(s) may not be identical for each animal affected. It is possible, therefore, that different treatments and preventive measures may be required for each case. However, until we understand the underlying pathophysiology of equine rhabdomyolysis, the treatment and prevention will remain empirical.

REFERENCES AND FURTHER READING

Arighi, M., Baird, J. D. & Hulland, T. J. (1984). *Compendium of Continuing Education for the Practising Veterinarian* **6(12)**, S726-S732.
Carlstrom, B. (1932). *Skandinavisches Archiv fur Physiologie* **63**, 164–212.
Fuji, Y., Watanabe, H., Yamamoto, T., Niwa, K., Muzuoka, S. & Anezaki, R. (1983). *Bulletin of the Equine Research Institute* **20**, 87–96.
Harris, P. (1988). Some aspects of the equine rhabdomyolysis syndrome. PhD thesis, Cambridge University.
Harris, P. A. & Colles, C. M. (1988). *Equine Veterinary Journal* **20**, 459–463.
Hodgson, D. R. (1985). *Compendium of Continuing Education for the Practising Veterinarian* **7(10)**, S551-S555.
Lindholm, A., Johansson, H. F. & Kjaersgaard, P. (1974). *Acta Veterinaria Scandanavia* **15**, 325–339.

McEwen, S. A. & Hulland, T. J. (1986). *Veterinary Pathology* **23**, 400–410.
McLean, J. G. (1973). *Australian Veterinary Journal* **49**, 41–43.
Waldron-Mease, E. (1979). *Journal of Equine Medicine and Surgery* **3**, 124–128.

CHAPTER 18

Assessment of Fitness in the Horse

DAVID SNOW

INTRODUCTION

The aim of any racehorse trainer, eventer, show-jumper or competitor at pony club level, is to be able to have their horses adequately fit so that they have a chance of competing successfully against other animals of equal standing. A further benefit in having a suitably fit animal is that the risk of fatigue related injuries is reduced.

As fitness is a relative term, fitness requirements will differ with the level and type of competition and the inherent ability of the horse. In some instances a horse with high inherent ability will not require the same degree of fitness as a lesser animal. Even some of the best horse experts have difficulty in judging when the appropriate stage of fitness has been reached. This is especially so for top class competition where there is a very fine line between peak fitness and overtraining, the latter leading to impaired performance.

AIMS OF A TRAINING PROGRAMME

Fitness is improved by adopting a training programme designed for the type of competition to be undertaken. Improvements aimed for are concerned with developments in the following areas:

(1) Improved energy production to better withstand fatigue. This involves adaptation both within the muscle fibres as aerobic capacity is increased, as well as a parallel change in the cardiovascular system to allow increased transport of oxygen to the muscle fibres.
(2) Structural changes in bones and tendons to better withstand the mechanical stress imposed during movement. Unfortunely little is presently known on this aspect.
(3) Improved skill brought about by the development of neuromuscular coordination.
(4) Psychological familiarity leading to the horse carrying out the task in a relaxed manner, which will lead to energy conservation.

Obviously all these factors are vital. Their relative importance, however, will vary for different types of competition. For example, improved energy production is very important over most racing distances and endurance events, while it is less so in show jumping and dressage, where neuromuscular coordination is of utmost importance. It is beyond the scope of this chapter to consider the specific training methods to attain the appropriate level of fitness. However, specificity is important when considering assessment of fitness, i.e. the training programme has to be developed for the particular type of competition and individualism. Each individual responds differently and therefore training programmes can only act as guidelines which need to be modified according to the response of the animal.

ASSESSMENT OF FITNESS

In considering the wider ramifications of fitness it is not sufficient merely to discuss assessment of improvements in the physiological and biochemical capacities of the horse. As shown in Table 18.1, mental and health aspects are also vital in ensuring optimum athletic performance.

FITNESS TESTS

In the past, assessment of fitness has been left to subjective evaluation by either the trainer and, or, the rider using various criteria. These may vary from trainer to trainer.

To overcome some of the problems inherent in subjective evaluation, a number of scientific tests, carried out under standardized conditions, have been devised to assess both stamina and strength in the human athlete. At the present time a number of research institutes are assessing the suitability of these for the horse. Tests under investigation are concerned with stamina. Such tests have a twofold function; first, to be able to assess an individual's fitness, and second, to be used in comparing the effectiveness of different training programmes.

Table 18.1 Important factors in fitness

Training effects
(1) Physiological and biochemical adaptations in:
   Muscle
   Cardiovascular
   Thermoregulation
(2) Structural strengthening in:
   Bone
   Tendon
(3) Skill – neuromuscular coordination
Behavioural
Health

OBSERVATION

The traditional method of assessment has relied on observing the animals, both at work and within the stable. The ability to observe is one of the important qualities in a good trainer. While at exercise the rider and, or, trainer will observe how the horse works, the day to day progress and overall performance in terms of expectations. Within racing yards the performance of several animals of similar ability are compared.

To help this assessment in some countries the racehorses' training gallops are timed. Interestingly this is rare in Great Britain.

Respiratory patterns are easily heard and observed and have, therefore, found extensive use in evaluating a horse's fitness. Clearly, the more unfit the horse, the longer the forceful respiration will continue after exercise. This increased respiration after exercise is due to the necessity for the horse to repay the oxygen deficit arising from lactic acid formation with high intensity exercise.

In endurance rides the measurement of respiratory rates is used at checkpoints as one of the criteria to judge whether a horse has sufficient fitness to continue. In Britain, if respiratory rates are twice the heart rate after a 30 min stop, the horse is eliminated. However, in America and Australia, although respiratory rates are noted, high rates do not result in the horse being eliminated, as it is realized that this can be elevated in the absence of fatigue when environmental temperatures are high. In hot climates, fast, shallow respiration is used as a means of heat dissipation. It is only when respiration is both frequent and deep that fatigue should be suspected and verified by an elevated heart rate.

WEIGHT

An important, but little used, aid in assessing fitness is the weight of the horse. Most horses come into training appreciably overweight and a reduction should occur as training progresses. Although it would appear obvious that an overweight horse, just as an overweight human, cannot perform at its best, it is surprising how many horses at both the racecourse and at other forms of competition are overweight.

The excuse for this is that the owner/trainer wants the horse to appear in good condition and not as skin and bones. However, it should be realized that an overweight horse is handicapped just as much as if it were carrying an overweight rider. This applies to any event that involves maximum effort, whether in a race or an endurance ride. This is because the more weight carried the more energy has to be expended per stride and, therefore, extra demands are made on what may already be overstretched energy supplying pathways. A justification put forward for having overweight horses compete in endurance rides is that fat is an important fuel for energy production. It should be realized, however, that even in a thin horse there are sufficient fat deposits to allow the horse to perform for days.

Although many trainers and riders feel that they can accurately estimate a horse's weight and feel insulted when challenged on this, the reality is that this is generally not possible and measurement methods should be used. Commercially available walk-on weigh-bridges are ideal. These are now used in a number of the larger thoroughbred racing stables. Alternatively, for those who cannot afford weigh-bridges, a number of measuring tapes are available to provide reasonably accurate measurements.

By regularly weighing horses, a number of the leading racing stables in this country have found that each horse has an ideal racing weight and anything above or below this weight may result in reduced performance. Perhaps surprisingly, a horse's ideal racing weight does not alter between its 2- and 3-year-old seasons. A slight gain may be seen when they are 4-year-olds.

STANDARDIZED EXERCISE TESTS

So that improved fitness can be properly quantified, standardized exercise tests have been developed. These include:

(1) Infield tests in which similar conditions are difficult to reproduce because of daily variations in factors such as track conditions, wind and the difficulty, especially for thoroughbreds, in maintaining constant speeds
(2) Tests using high-speed treadmills preferably in a controlled environment.

In these tests, both physiological and biochemical parameters can be measured either during or following workloads of fixed intensity and duration. At present the most common physiological parameter measured is heart rate, while blood samples are collected on which numerous biochemical assays can be carried out. For fitness assessment, these tests are presently confined to blood lactate measurements and some enzymes.

Although many people may think that working horses on highspeed treadmills is dangerous and unnatural, experience over 20 years in Sweden, and now in other institutes throughout the world, has shown that horses work readily and safely on them. With the high speed treadmills that have come on to the market within the last year, racing conditions can be simulated when horses are galloped or trotted on them. Having horses working on these not only allows more standardized conditions, but also allows easier monitoring during the exercise period itself (Fig. 18.1). Not only will treadmills find greater use in fitness testing, but they should also be of great assistance in assessing clinical disorders that are only apparent at exercise.

AEROBIC CAPACITY

Increasing stamina depends on the development of the horse's aerobic capacity which is reflected by changes at the muscle fibre level, leading to increased activity of enzymes involved

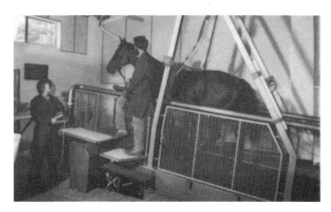

Fig. 18.1
Horse exercising on a treadmill.

in oxidative metabolism and increased numbers of capillaries surrounding the fibres (Fig. 18.2). This in turn increases the anaerobic threshold, so that higher speeds can be undertaken without risk of lactate related fatigue occurring. In addition, the metabolic changes within muscle also allow the proportion of fat to glucose utilized to increase, an important factor in preventing fatigue in endurance activities, as in this case glycogen depletion is the cause of fatigue. A number of methods of varying complexities have been developed to measure any improvement in aerobic capacity.

Oxygen consumption

In man, one of the oldest methods of measuring improved aerobic capacity was to measure changes in maximal oxygen consumption (VO_2max) during the training programme. However, this test is not used as frequently today, because major differences between individuals are genetically determined, with only small increases occurring within an individual with training, despite obvious increases in fitness. In horses, determination of oxygen consumption is possible, but the technique is only in its infancy and although horses tolerate wearing the masks required for the tests, it is unlikely that

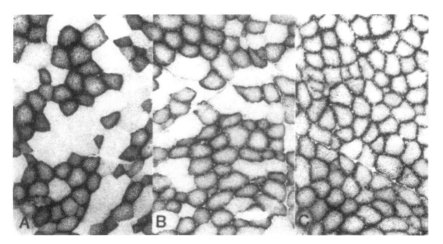

Fig. 18.2 Change in oxidative capacity of fibres in thoroughbred racehorses with training. (A) Early training; (B) end of first year of training; (C) end of second year of training.

this will develop as a routine fitness test. In the horse, VO_2max is of the order of 140–150 ml/kg/min, compared to elite human athletes of 80 ml/kg/min. It is more likely that tests associated with gaseous exchange will develop to evaluate functional disturbances related to respiratory disease.

Anaerobic threshold

The determination of anaerobic threshold, also referred to as the onset of blood lactate accumulation, involves finding the work intensity at which there is a sudden upsurge in the blood lactic acid concentration, i.e. the point at which production is not matched by the rate of removal from the blood. The anaerobic threshold is determined by working the horse at a number of speeds for 2 or 3 min per workload and taking blood samples each time for lactate measurement. The results are then plotted on a graph and the anaerobic threshold determined (Fig. 18.3). For ease of calculation, the concentration above which blood lactate is said to be raised has been arbitrarily set at 4 mmol/litre.

In man there is a close correlation between anaerobic threshold and performance in marathon races. Therefore, this should be a very good test to assess an endurance horse's

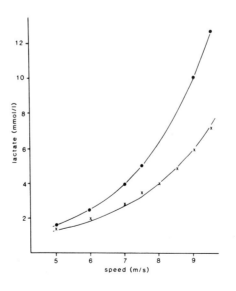

Fig. 18.3
Change in anaerobic threshold with training. (Modified from Thornton et al., 1983). ●, Before training; x, after training.

ability to perform. With shorter events the correlation to performance is not as good and for sprinting events of around one minute duration it may have only limited value. This is because as oxidative capacity within muscle fibres (and therefore anaerobic threshold) is increased, the muscle fibres may become smaller in size so that the ability of the muscle to produce power is reduced. In other words, both stamina and strength cannot be developed optimally at the same time.

At the present time a number of research groups are trying to evaluate the anaerobic threshold test as a means of assessing fitness and performance ability in horses. These tests involve either exercising the horse on a treadmill for periods of 2 min at progressively increasing speeds, or they can be exercised over 1000 metres at each of four different speeds. Standardized speeds of 450–500, 600–700, 700–800 and greater than 800 metres per minute have been used, with blood samples for lactate estimations being collected after three minutes at each speed.

Heart rate

Of all the objective means of assessing fitness, monitoring the heart rate is the easiest and can be readily carried out by most riders. For this purpose a number of onboard heart rate meters are commercially available. Unfortunately, not all are reliable, especially at high workloads. Two meters found to be accurate are the Equistat (EQB, Unionville, USA), shown in Figure 18.4, and the Hippocard (Polar Electro, Finland). Each costs in the region of £500. They provide heart rate readings via a digital display. Later models of the Hippocard contain a memory chip which allows data to be recorded and recalled later. The latest version of the Hippocard (Sport Tester, PE 3000) allows a permanent record of the data, as it can be transferred via a computer to a printer (Fig. 18.5).

When horses are worked at the same effort and the same level of fitness, very reproducible heart rates are seen. Using increasing workloads it has been shown that heart rates increase linearly with effort between 120 and 210 beats per minute. Above this level there is a gradual plateauing, although in young animals maximal heart rates as high as 250 beats per minute can be attained at maximum effort. As horses

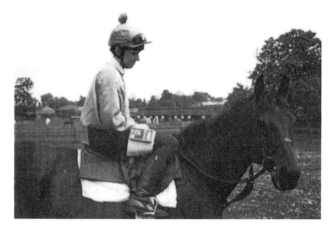

Fig. 18.4
On board heart rate
meter (EQB model).

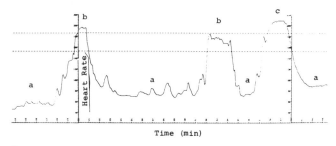

Time (min)

Fig. 18.5 Computer print out from an on board heart rate meter (Hippocard model). a, Walk; b, canter; c, gallop.

become fitter both the resting and working heart rates become lower, with rates as low as 25 beats per minute at rest. At low workloads and during recovery, the heart rate can be influenced by external stimuli, inasmuch as a heart rate can momentarily jump from 120 to 180 beats per minute if the horse is startled.

It has been suggested that one method of assessing fitness is to find the work intensity required to cause a heart rate of 200 beats per minute. For example, using this criterion in standardbreds it was found that 5 weeks of training had increased the speed to cause a heart rate of 200 beats/min from 7·35 to 7·96 m/s on a treadmill at a 10° incline.

In addition to monitoring heart rates during exercise, it has also been found useful to measure them during the recovery period. Following exercise the most rapid fall in heart rate occurs in the first few minutes. When using recovery heart rates to assess fitness, it has been found that the five-minute rate is the most useful after exercise, and obviously should be lower following a similar exercise as the horse becomes fitter.

It has also been suggested that daily monitoring of heart rates at exercise can provide an early warning sign of health problems. For example, it has been found that lameness can cause elevations above the expected heart rates, even before the lameness becomes visible.

Enzymes

The monitoring of enzymes that may indicate muscle damage can also be useful in assessing fitness in racehorses. In the early stages of training when heavier workloads are first introduced, elevations in the plasma activities of creatine phosphokinase (CPK) and aspartate aminotransferase (AST, GOT, AAT) often recur because of muscle damage. With increasing fitness these elevations usually disappear following exercise until, in the fit animal, remarkably constant values are seen week after week. When this stage is reached, even a small increase in enzyme activities should be investigated as potentially significant. In endurance horses it has been found that some horses can compete successfully with quite marked plasma elevations in these enzymes. Another plasma enzyme worthy of monitoring is γ-glutamyl transferase (GGT) and this will be discussed below.

Often veterinary surgeons are called in when horses are performing below expectations. This can either be real, when performance is below previous efforts, or because the high expectations of the owner are not being met. It can then be very difficult to decide whether such performances are caused by lack of fitness, general changes in management procedures or a health problem. The difficulties in assessing the state of fitness properly have been discussed and the chapter will conclude by considering briefly some tests that may be of assistance in assessing health problems in competition animals. These are of help when below par performance is not associated with any other clinical signs at rest.

ASSESSMENT OF HEALTH

Hand in hand with an adequate training programme to attain peak fitness is the requirement for optimum health of a horse. This involves the correct management procedures, such as regular worming, dental and foot care, vaccination and housing in well ventilated stables. Health problems will cause setbacks in training, as well as leading to disappointment on the day of competition. To ensure a healthy horse and the early detection of minor problems, needs a trainer/owner to observe carefully the horse at work and at rest.

In association with the normal surveillance by a veterinary surgeon, a number of racehorse trainers have routine blood tests carried out on their horses. Although, fortunately, in the majority of cases these show that the horse is perfectly normal, it is the belief of the author that if regularly taken they can provide an early warning that all may not be well with an individual horse, or that there is a problem within the stable. If blood monitoring is to be most effective, samples should be collected before the commencement of training and then monthly during the training season. This allows the normal baseline values for each individual to be established so that the significance of minor deviations can be assessed. It is also important that samples are collected at a consistent time. Ideally, they should be collected in the morning before feeding and exercise. However, if this is not possible, then at evening stables on a day when only light exercise has been given.

Both the cellular and plasma fractions of blood are examined. Total white cell counts and differentials are considered extremely valuable, in that they can provide an indication of both clinical and subclinical disease problems. In the author's opinion, monitoring of red blood cell parameters is of lesser value. The occurrence of a true anaemia is extremely rare, although depressed haematocrits and red blood cell counts are often seen in association with viral and other diseases. A return to normal values is seen as the horse recovers.

The usefulness of measuring plasma CPK and AST activities has already been mentioned. As well as its possible place in aiding measurement of fitness, it is also of use in determining the severity of suspected cases of rhabdomyolysis (tying-up, setfast, azoturia). Recently, studies at the Animal Health Trust have indicated that the measurement of plasma GGT may be extremely useful in assessing whether a horse has been over-stressed during training. With training there is often a gradual rise in plasma GGT activity.

Why this occurs is unknown but it would appear to be a normal response to the stress of training. However, in some animals activities can rise to above 100 iu (the normal range within the Animal Health Trust laboratory is up to 50 iu). When this occurs racing performances below expectations can be seen, especially if the enzyme activity continues to rise. In such cases, the horse should be carefully examined for any minor problems as it is found that these horses will appear normal at rest, perform well in training gallops, but will fade under the demands made for maximal effort during racing. If strenuous exercise is undertaken in horses with lower or upper respiratory problems a rise in GGT may occur. Once the problem has been resolved, or the stress imposed by training is reduced, only a gradual decline in plasma activity of this enzyme occurs as it has a plasma half-life of over 2 weeks. An example of plasma GGT activities in two thorough-bred fillies during two racing seasons is shown in Figure 18.6.

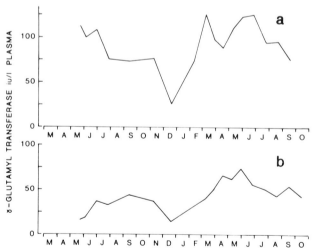

Fig. 18.6 Plasma γ-glutamyl transferase activities during two racing seasons in the thoroughbred fillies. (a) Horse with high activity and a performance below expectations. (b) Fluctuations that may occur during a season.

Index

"2-year-old squeak", 152

Abdominal haemorrhage, 99
Abscess, 217
  intra-abdominal, 123
Acepromazine, 200, 275
Acidosis, 278
Adequan, 204, 209
Adrenalin, 31, 212
Aerobic capacity, 286–287
Air filters, 68
Air hygiene, 59 ff
Air samplers, 69
Airborne particle counter, 63
Alkalosis, 272, 276
Ammonia, 60, 76
Ampicillin, 13
Anaemia, 153
Anaerobic threshold, 288–289
Animalintex, 186
Antebrachium, 261
Anterior enteritis, 99, 120
Anthracoides spp., 10
Aorta, 116–117
Aortic incompetence, 145
Aortic stenosis, 145
Artificial insemination, 17
Aspergillus fumigatus, 70
Ataxia, 23
Atresia, 139
Atrial fibrillation, 147 ff, 155 ff, 158

Atrial septal defect, 148
Atrioventricular heart block, 147–148,
  156
Aureomycin, 187
Azoturia, 292

Bacteroides fragilis, 11, 13
Bedding, 70, 76–77
"Bench knee", 164
Benzylpenicillin, 13
Blepharospasm, 131
Botulism, 76
"Breathing roof", 67
Bronchoscopy, 84
Bruising, 217, 220
Bupivacaine, 201
Butorphanol, 30

Caecal intussusception, 121
Caecum, 118
Calcium carbonate, 200
Calculi, 20, 22
Cannula, 137 ff
  indwelling, 138
Carbocaine, 213
Carbohydrate overloading, 272
Cardiology, clinical aspects, 143 ff
Carpal tunnel syndrome, 225
Carpus, 258 ff
Caslick's vulvoplasty, 4–5, 27 ff

Catheter
  Foley, 16
  indwelling uterine infuser, 13–14
  urethral, 22
  see also Cannula
Cauda equina neuritis, 20, 23
Cellulitis, 167
Cervical damage, 7–8, 14, 16
Cervicitis, 3 ff, 7, 28, 30
Cetavlex, 198
Chip fracture, 247
Chlortetracycline, 187
Chorionic gonadotrophin stimulation
  test, 42
Chronic obstructive pulmonary disease,
  148
Chronic pulmonary disease, 59 ff
Citanest, 213
Clicks, 148–149
Clostridium mortiferum, 11
Clostridium perfringens, 11
Colic, 56, 99, 101, 267
Colon, blocked, 119
  large, 118
  large: entrapment, 121–122
  small, 118–119
Colonic displacement, 119, 123
Colonic obstruction, 123
Colonic stasis, 119–120
Colonic torsion, 119, 123, 128
Corns, 172–173, 189 ff
Corticosteroids, 197–198, 205, 275–276
Corynebacterium spp., 10
Coughing, 62
Cracked heels, 197–198
Cryptorchidectomy, 42 ff
Cryptorchidism, 41 ff
Crystapen, 13
Cyanosis, 82, 144
Cystitis, 20 ff

Dacryocystorhinography, 135
Dantrolene, 275, 277–278
Degenerative joint disease, 203
Dermobion, 198
Desmitis, 177, 217, 223
Desmotomy, 197
Detomidine hydrochloride, 30, 137
Diarrhoea, 38

Diazepam, 275
Digoxin, 159
Dimethylglycine, 277–278
Discharge, urinary tract, 2
  vaginal, 1 ff
Distal phalanx, 244 ff
  fracture, 201 ff, 217, 220, 234
Distal sesamoid bone, 249 ff
Domosedan, 30, 137
Draughts, 64–65
"Dup" sound, 147–148
Ductus arteriosus, patent, 153
Dust mites, 60
Dyspnoea, 59
Dystocia, 8

Electrolyte solution, 276 ff
Emaciation, 101
Endocarditis, 144
Endometritis, 2, 4–5, 7 ff, 24, 28, 30, 37
Enteritis, 123
Enterobacter aerogenes, 11
Enzymes: in fitness monitoring, 291
Epidydimis, 47 ff
Escherichia coli, 4, 10
Ethmoid haematoma, 84
Exercise tests, 285–286

Facial paralysis, bilateral, 84
Fetlock, 253 ff
  sprain, 205
Fibrosis, periarticular, 237
Finadyne, 199
Fitness assessment, 281 ff
Flexion tests, 175
Flexor tendon, 168–169
  strain, 208 ff
Flexor tendonitis, 217
Flunixine meglumine, 199, 275
Fluorescein dye, 140
Foot: pus in, 185 ff, 239
Forearm, 261
Frusemide, 20
Fucidin-H, 15
Fungal spore clouds, 60, 62
Furaltadone, 13

Gastric dilatation, 99

Gastroduodenitis, 120
Gastrointestinal tract, 115
Glycosaminoglycan, 204
Glycosaminoglycan polysulphate,
    208–209
Gonadotrophin, human, 42
Grass sickness, 97 ff, 120
Gut infarction, 128

Haemorrhage
    abdominal, 99
    nasal, 113
    vaginal, 3
Health assessment, 292–293
Heart, 143 ff
    auscultation, 145
    rate, 155, 289 ff
    rhythm, 155–156
    sounds, 146 ff
Helminthiasis, 99
Herpesvirus-1, 20, 23, 61
Hock, 262
Hoof testers, 172–173
Hydrocortisone, 15
Hydrocortisone acidate, 15
Hydrogen peroxide, 186, 192
Hylartil, 206
Hypertension, 200
Hyperthermia, 274, 278
Hypothermia, 64
Hypothyroidism, 273
Hypovolaemia, 120
Hypoxia, 272

Incontinence
    overflow, 23
    urinary, 20
Inguinal herniation, 118
Intra Epicaine, 213
Intra-articular anaesthesia, 231 ff
Intra-articular analgesia, 228 ff
Iodine, 192
Ionizers, 68
Isoxsuprine, 195

Joint capsule distension, 170

Keratoma, 220
Kidney, 117
Klebsiella pneumoniae, 11, 31

Lameness
    diagnosis, 211 ff
    diagnosis, use of intra-articular
        anaesthesia in, 231 ff
    forelimb: diagnosis, 161 ff
    intermittent, 240
Laminitis, 162, 169, 172, 174, 180, 198 ff,
    220, 239
Large intestine
    distension, 121
    herniation, 99
    impaction, 99
    infarction, 99
    obstruction, 99
    volvulus, 99
Laryngeal paralysis, 82, 85
Lectade, 276
Leg swellings, 166–167
Lignocaine, 212
Lignocaine hydrochloride, 31, 137
Limb: anatomy, 243 ff
Lower Respiratory Tract Inflammation,
    60
"Lubb" sound, 147

Mating: after Caslick's vulvoplasty, 35
Mating techniques, minimal
        contamination, 17–18
Meclofenamic acid, 275
Meglumine iothalamate, 135
Mepivacaine, 213
Mesenteric root, 117
Mesocolon, 119
Metacarpal/metatarsal bones, 255 ff
Metacarpophalangeal/metatarsophalangeal
        joint, 253 ff
Methadone, 275
Methionine, 200
Methocarbamol, 275
Metronidazole, 187–188
Middle phalanx, 251
Mitral incompetence, 153
Mitral insufficiency, 144
"Monday morning" disease, 265

Murmurs, 149 ff
  continuous, 153
  diastolic, 152
  systolic, 150 ff
Muscle atrophy, 163–164
Myocarditis, 158
Myoglobinuria, 267

Nail bind or prick, 191–192
Nasal haemorrhage, 113
Nasogastric intubation, 107 ff, 127
Nasolacrimal cannulation, 135 ff
Navicular bone fracture, 217, 234
Navicular disease, 162 ff, 169, 173–174,
    179, 192 ff, 217, 232 ff
Neomycin, 13, 188
Neoplasia, intra-abdominal, 123
  nasal, 84
Nephritis, 99
Nephrosplenic ligament, 117, 121–122
Nerve block, 211 ff
  auriculopalpebral and palpebral,
    131 ff
  medial, 223 ff
  palmar, 179, 201, 203, 217
  palmar and palmar metacarpal,
    221–222
  palmar digital, 217, 239
  sub-carpal, 222–223
  ulnar, 223 ff
Neurectomy, palmar digital, 196

Ophthaine, 137
Ossification, 247 ff, 256
Osteitis, 183, 189
Osteoarthrosis, 165
Osteochondrosis, 174, 262
Osteomyelitis, 189
Osteophytes, 264
Overweight, 284–285
Oxygen consumption, 287–288
Oxytetracycline, 188

Pain, joint, 240
Paracentesis, 127
Paralysis, radial nerve, 163
Paresis, 23
Parturition: after Caslick's vulvoplasty,
    35

Pastern bones, 251 ff
Pedal bone: wing fracture, 172
Pelvis, 116–117
Penicillin, 13, 56
Peptococcus spp., 11
Peptostreptococcus spp., 11
Periostitis, 207
Peritoneum, 119
Peritonitis, 56, 99, 122
Pethidine hydrochloride, 56
Phenothiazine, 275, 277
Phenylbutazone, 173, 194, 199, 204–205,
    216, 275
Placental separation, 3, 19
Placentitis, 18
Pneumouterus, 4
Pneumovagina, 1, 3, 7, 14, 18, 27 ff
Polymixin, 13
Polyps, 20, 23
Post injection reaction, 82
Potassium chloride, 200
Poultice, 186–187, 192, 216
Pouret's perineal reconstruction, 6
Prednisolone, 198
Premature beats, 147, 157–158
Prilocaine, 213
Procaine penicillin G, 187
Prostaglandins, 15
Proteus spp., 11
Proximal phalanx, 251 ff
Proximal sesamoid bone fracture, 237
Proxymetacaine hydrochloride, 137–138
Pseudomonas aeruginosa, 11, 13, 16, 31
Pulmonary stenosis, 153
Pyometra, 7, 15–16, 24

Quinidine gluconate, 159
Quinidine intoxication, 158
Quinidine sulphate, 159

Radial nerve paralysis, 163
Radiography
  in lameness, 179 ff
  limb, 243 ff
Rectal examination of the
    gastrointestinal tract, 115
Rectal rupture, 128–129
Rectovaginal damage, 8, 14
Respiratory disease, 59 ff

Respiratory obstruction, 82
Respiratory patterns, 284
Rhabdomyolysis, 265 ff
Rhinovirus-1, 61
Ringbone, 169–170, 203
Rugs: insulating material used as, 64

Salmonellosis, 123
Scopulariopsis brevicaulis, 70
Seedy toe, 220
Selenium, 275 ff
Selenium deficiency, 273
Semen extenders, 17
Septicaemia, 158
Sesamoiditis, 222
Setfast, 292
Shoe: removal, 178
Shoeing, 165–166
    problems, 217, 220
Sidebone, 169–170
Small intestine
    distension, 120
    impaction, 120, 123
    infarction, 120
    intussusception, 120
    muscular hypertrophy, 122
    obstruction, 99, 120
Sodium bicarbonate, 275–276
Sodium chloride, 200
Sodium fusidate, 15
Sodium hyaluronate, 204, 206
Sodium salicylate, 277
Soft palate subluxation, 85
Spleen, 117–118
"Splints", 164, 207–208, 223, 235–236
Sprain: fetlock, 206
Staphylococcus albus, 4, 10
Staphylococcus aureus, 4, 10
Stifle, 262
Stings, 82
Stomach pump, *see* Nasogastric
    intubation
Strain: flexor tendon, 208 ff
Streptococcus faecalis, 11
Streptococcus zooepidemicus, 4, 10
Subchondral bone cyst, 220, 225, 235
Subchondral bone sclerosis, 204
Sulphanilamide, 31, 198
Sulphur hexafluoride, 63

"Sunken" anus, 28
Supra-pubic paramedian laparotomy,
    50 ff, 56–57
Suture line breakdown, 37–38

Tachycardia, 147, 155, 158–159
Tarsus, 262
Taylorella equigenitalis, 11
Tendonitis, 223
Tenosynovitis, 223
Testes, non-descended, *see*
    Cryptorchidism
Testosterone, 42, 55
Tetracycline, 13
Thiamin, 275, 277–278
Thrill, 154–155
Thromboembolic colic, 99
Thrush, 217
Thyroxine, 277–278
Torbugesic, 30
Torgyl, 187
Toxaemia, 158
Tracheal obstruction, 85
Tracheostomy, 81 ff
    permanent, 82, 84 ff, 89 ff, 92 ff
    temporary, 81 ff, 89, 91–92
    tube cleaning, 94–95
Treadmills, 285–286
Tricuspid valve, incompetent, 144
Tumours, vesicular, 20, 23
Tying-up, 292

Ultrasound, 15, 23, 182–183
Underrun sole, 185 ff
Ureter, ectopic, 19
Urethritis, 20
Urinary tract
    abnormalities, 1
    discharge, 2
Urovagina, 28, 39
Uterine defence mechanisms, failure, 14
Uterine infuser, indwelling, 13–14
Uterine irrigation, 16–17
Uterus, gravid, 116

Vagina: faecal contamination, 28–29
Vaginal discharge, 1 ff
Vaginal haemorrhage, 3

Vaginal urine pooling, 18, 24
Vaginitis, 3 ff, 7, 18, 28
Varicose veins
  vaginal, 3
  vestibular, 19
Ventilation of buildings, 62 ff
Ventricular septal defect, 153
Verminous arteritis, 99
Vesicular endoscopy, 22

Vitamin E, 275 ff
Vulval conformation, concave, 39

Warfarin, 196

Xylazine, 115, 213, 275
Xylocaine, 137
Xylotox, 31